# TRISHA'S
## 21-DAY RESET

# TRISHA'S
## 21-DAY RESET

**3 WEEKS TO KICK-START YOUR WEIGHT-LOSS JOURNEY**

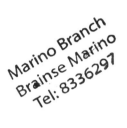

## TRISHA LEWIS
### GILL BOOKS

Gill Books

Hume Avenue

Park West

Dublin 12

www.gillbooks.ie

Gill Books is an imprint of M.H. Gill and Co.

9780 717190881

Designed by Jane Matthews

Portrait photography by Leo Byrne

Food photography by Joanne Murphy

Food styling by Orla Neligan

Edited by Kristin Jensen

Proofread by Emma Dunne

Nutritional information provided by Mary Daly Food Safety Company

Indexed by Adam Pozner

Printed by Printer Trento, Italy

This book is typeset in Neutraface

5 4 3 2

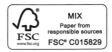

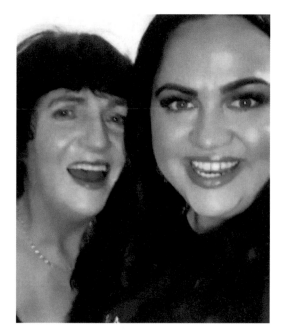

This book is for you, Mam. Nothing has changed since the first book
– you are still my hero.

Thank you for making me see what you always saw in me. You never once
gave up on me. All that I am and all that I dream to be is because of you.
Will you just admit that I am the favourite daughter so we can put the rest
of them out of their confusion?

# ABOUT THE AUTHOR

One of nine girls, 33-year-old Trisha Lewis grew up on a dairy farm in County Limerick. She studied Professional Cookery in CIT and for 13 years worked as the executive head chef of Jacobs on the Mall. In 2017 Trisha weighed in for a gastric bypass. She was 27 stone. She later cancelled the bypass, and then in 2018 she tipped the scales at 26 stone. At 25 stone, Trisha made the decision to document her weight-loss journey in the most public way possible by starting an Instagram page. She now has 187,000 followers, whom she lovingly calls her Transformers. In 2020, due to the Covid-19 pandemic, Trisha was let go from work and ended up gaining two stone. But, in true Transformer style, she decided to tackle this new challenge and has since changed her career and lost the weight she gained. And, after a lot of self-reflection, Trisha realised she needed extra help for her binge eating disorder and joined therapy. Now eight stone lighter, Trisha has given up smoking and is the happiest she has ever been. In this book Trisha shares the tools that have helped keep her on the road to happiness and lose weight in a sustainable and positive way. She hopes that with this book you too can find the belief inside yourself to truly change your life and beat the bulge.

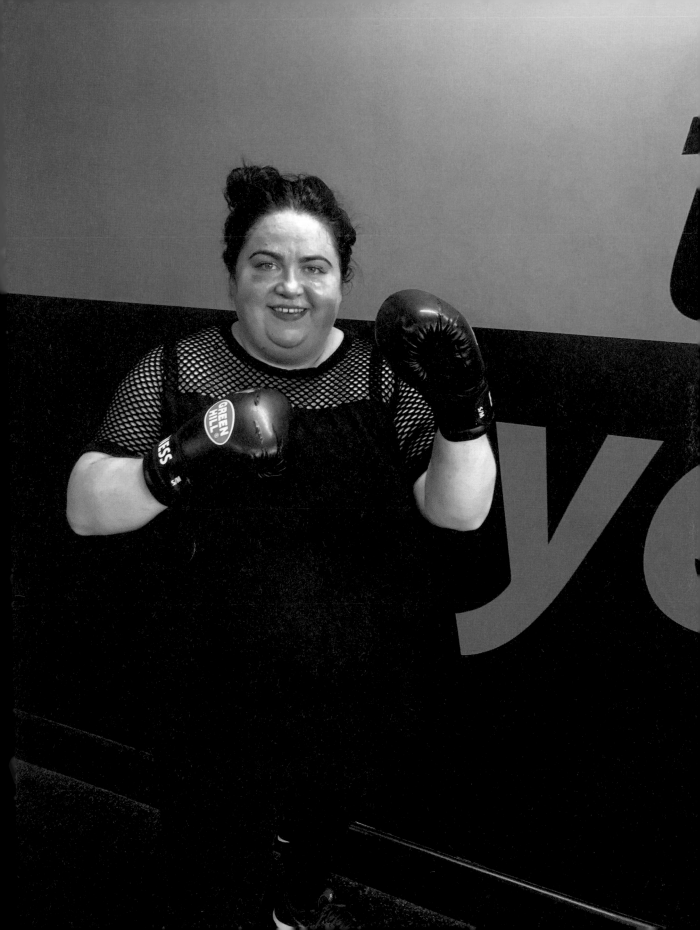

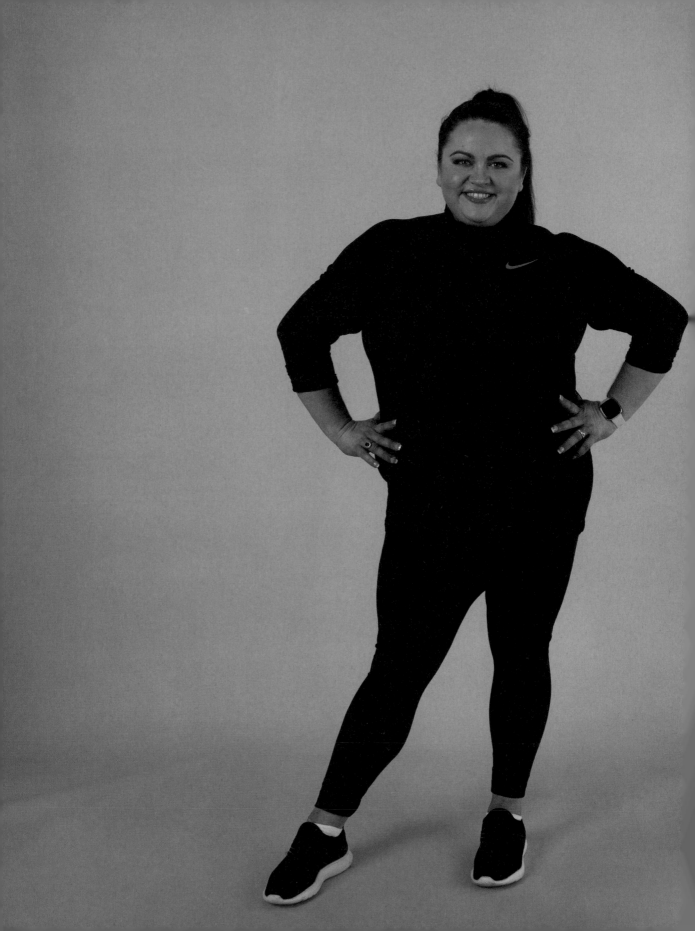

# CONTENTS

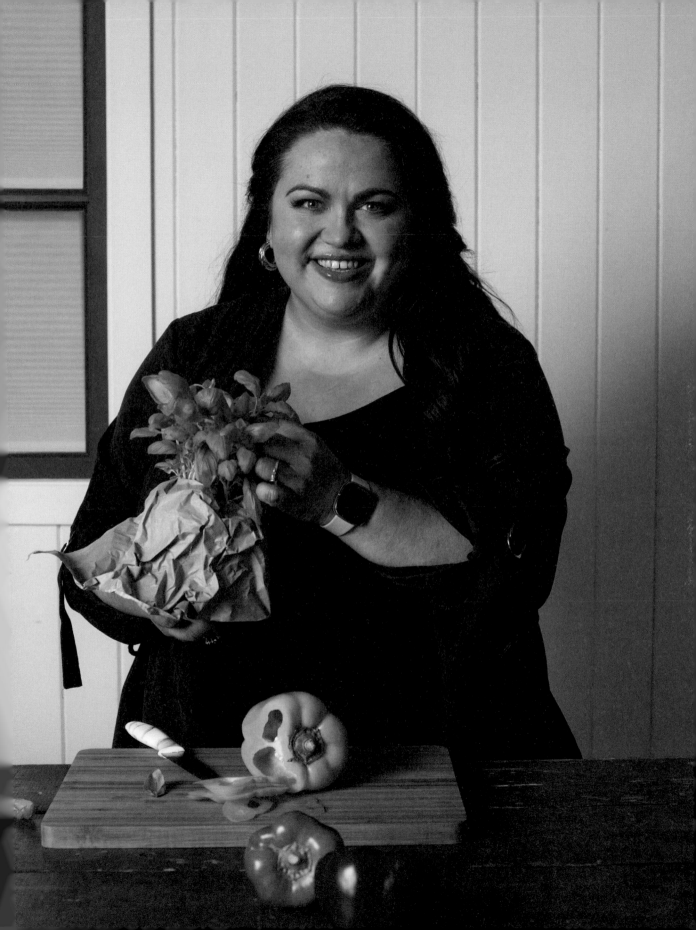

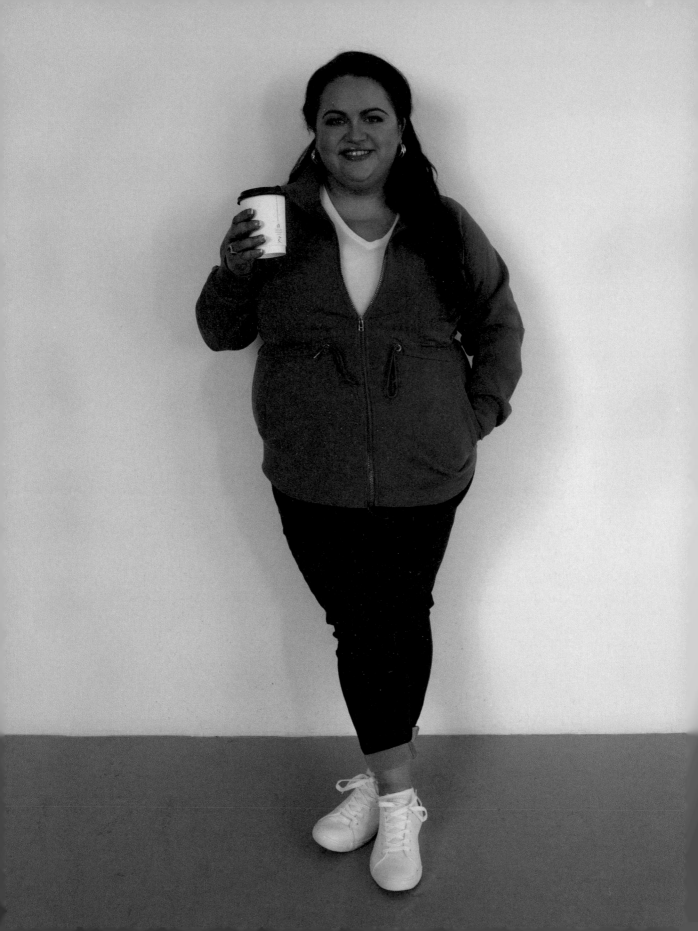

# INTRODUCTION

Hello, my Transformers! How are you getting on? Or if you're a new reader, I would like to introduce myself. My name is Trisha Lewis and I am on a mission to change my life and shed 13 stone – I'm over halfway there! I have been a trained chef for 13 years and was executive head chef at my beloved Jacobs on the Mall until August 2020, when I took a big scary leap and finished to follow a new dream. I am a true believer in amazing food, creating recipes for everyone and losing weight without losing flavour. I document my whole journey for my Transformers on my Instagram page, @trishas.transformation.

I can't believe that as I'm sitting here in October 2020, the wind is howling, we have just landed into a second lockdown and I am writing my second book. The months have flown by since I started to write this book. It's surreal, to say the least.

The reaction to my first book blew me away. If you'd told me when I was writing it in 2019 that every bookstore in Ireland would be closed by the time it was published due to the COVID-19 pandemic, I wouldn't have believed you. And yet it was the overall number 1 book in the country for one week and number 1 in paperback non-fiction for four weeks. The feedback to my first book has been everything that I dreamed it would be. People loved the simplicity and the flavour of my dishes. People laughed with me and cried with me. It reached the people who I wanted it to reach, the ones who had felt that they were alone in feeling desperate, lonely, sad and laughed at. The words hope, joy, faith and love bounced off the messages in my inbox and I could feel the drive that had been instilled in people.

My first book was all about me, my journey and my story. This book is for you. I want you to start your journey or use this book if you feel that you have fallen off the wagon. Everything that I know that has brought me on this 7.5 stone weight-loss journey is in this book so that you can learn from it. I don't have big words to explain how I feel and how I do it, so I will explain it to you in my own way. I have found this hard but also so enjoyable because I have taught myself resilience, and I put all that down to the power of resetting and giving myself 21 days of a system. I always know that by the end I will be feeling amazing and that I will have got tougher and more ready for the next time a curveball comes.

For this book all the calories and macros have been done for you, so it's for everyone, whether your goal is weight loss, healthy eating, shredding or whatever it may be. Diet food is simply food, and food is simply wonderful. It keeps us alive every single day and we should celebrate it and enjoy it instead of being miserable and dreaming of the Chinese take-away that you want to have. This book is packed full of dinners, breakfasts, fake-aways and snacks for you to enjoy.

Weight loss doesn't have to be negative. I spent all my adult life hating and avoiding the fact that I had to lose weight. I cried many times, feeling trapped because I felt like a failure. But I wasn't a failure – I just didn't have the correct systems in place. Now when things go wrong I don't beat myself up, I simply reset.

It's all about how you look at the glass: is it half full or is it half empty? I decided very early on that I would love my journey and that I would learn to love myself. Part of my journey is setbacks and curveballs, and if I love the good, then I also have to love and learn from the not-so-good parts. Part of a weight-loss journey inevitably involves weight gain at some stage, so how do I stay on track and keep going? By having the tools that this book is based on.

The diet culture is everywhere and success story after success story is pouring from our devices, but what happens when you feel like you've messed up and can't go on? What happens when you have a night out filled with wine and a bag of chips? What happens when you haven't slept well and all you want to do is pick the leftover food from your kids' plates? What happens when you're upset and have eaten extra calories and you feel like the only person in the world who does this? What happens when you are doing amazing and then all of a sudden you're tired and find yourself in the drive-through ordering food for a fake friend? (I've ordered food for 'Mary' so many times, but in fact it was all for me.) What happens when you feel like you're bogged down and you just can't get your mojo back?

The answer is, you RESET.

This book will guide you for three weeks. If you follow the guidelines for three weeks, you will feel better. You will feel like you are back in control. All of us 'mess up', but one thing I've learned from my journey is that you need to be resilient and resilience comes from never giving up, no matter what your mind is telling you, no matter what the scales say. You hold the power because you are the boss of your own happiness.

We can often overthink things, but I am hoping that this book will help you to see that the simplest things are the most important. So get the basics right. Go for the low-hanging fruit.

I want you to commit to making the next three weeks the most important three weeks of your life. After every single round of three weeks, simply reset and repeat what you did the previous three weeks if it made you feel good. Feeling like crap is just feedback that you are not giving yourself the chance that you need.

In this book I will talk you through establishing the foundation for a complete reset. I want you to do the 21-day reset 17 times this year and I want you to really smash it. You are well able to do it!

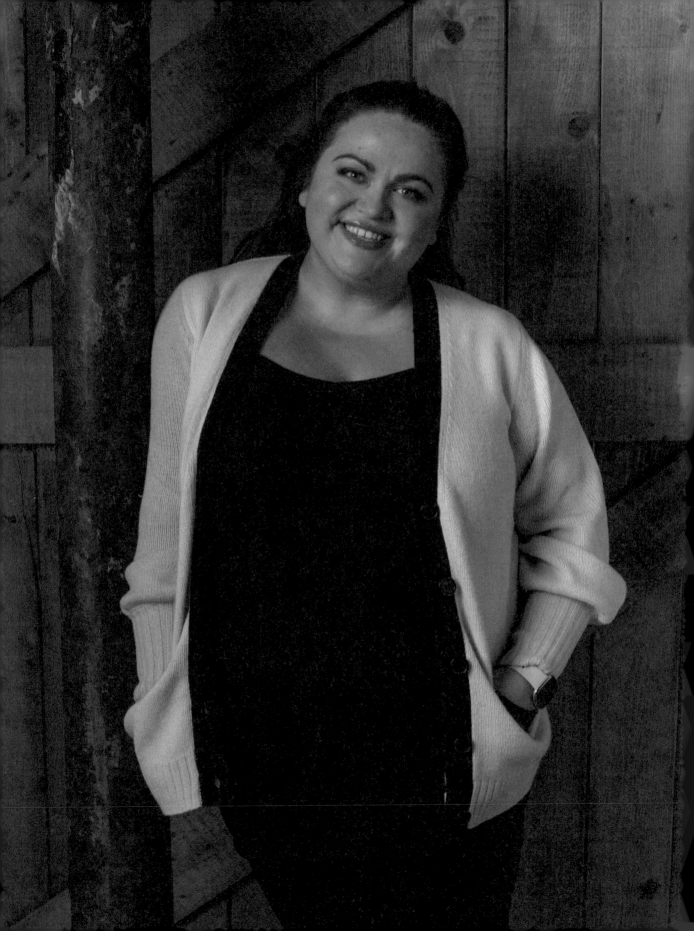

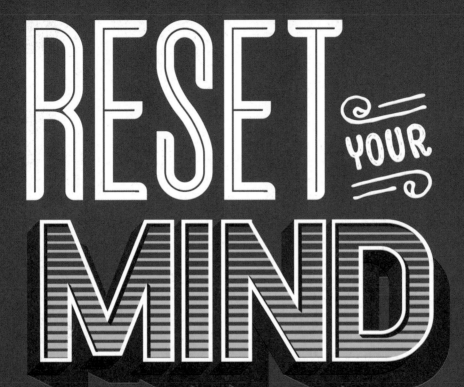

# FAILURE IS POSITIVE

I often get asked what to do after you've hit the self-sabotage button, and the answer is reset. Failure will happen – this is not going to be plain sailing. The negative feedback that you may have got all your life might mean that you feel useless and unable to achieve a healthy lifestyle. But let's flip all that around now and look at failure as a positive thing. In a weird way, failure is a gift because it's a warning shot that your system isn't working and that you need to reset.

Stop beating yourself up that when you went into a garage to pay for your petrol, you bought four KitKats too. You're human. It happens. Instead of following this up with self-hate and throwing your whole journey out the window, take a deep breath and say, 'Right, that happened. I can't undo it, but it doesn't make me a bad person, just a person who went into a garage when I was hungry and went a bit mad.' When this happens, make a plan based on what went wrong before. I have a rule with garages that I abide by about 90% of the time. I call it the diesel diet. I will only purchase diesel because it's too easy to sit in the car at the pumps afterwards, scoff down the food and put the wrappers in the bin.

As I explained in my first book, the lightbulb moment is fleeting. Things will slowly get brighter, but you have to work on it bit by bit, plan by plan. You have to keep resetting. Over time, resetting when things get hard will get easier and easier.

Armed with the knowledge that failure will happen, you can be ready for it with a smile and the best tool in the toolbox: the reset. Your inner critic won't expect positivity, so catch it off guard and watch how much easier life is when your mind doesn't go to the negative side straight away. How you react to and deal with failure will determine your journey.

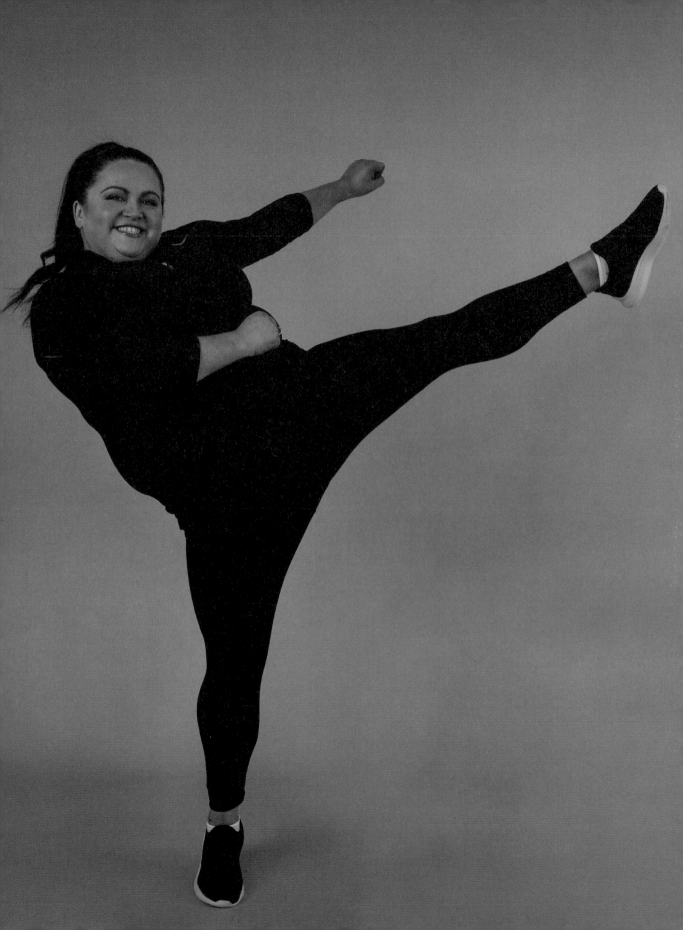

# FIND YOUR WHY

I know that you are hurting, that you have been hurt by others and mainly that you have hurt yourself by how you think of yourself. I know that you are tired. You are sick of failing and sick of never being the person you have always dreamed you can be. I know all of that, but I also know that you are capable, that you are strong and that you can do this.

Before you can play this ace card that is the reset button in your everyday life, let's look at a very important question. This question will be your guide every time you need to change course.

Every book I read and every podcast that I listen to says over and over again that you need to find your why:

**Why am I doing this?**

..................................................................................................................

..................................................................................................................

..................................................................................................................

..................................................................................................................

..................................................................................................................

My why keeps changing. I have new goals and I adjust as I go, but my main why will always be that I want to be happy. I want to go to sleep without crying. I want to feel healthy.

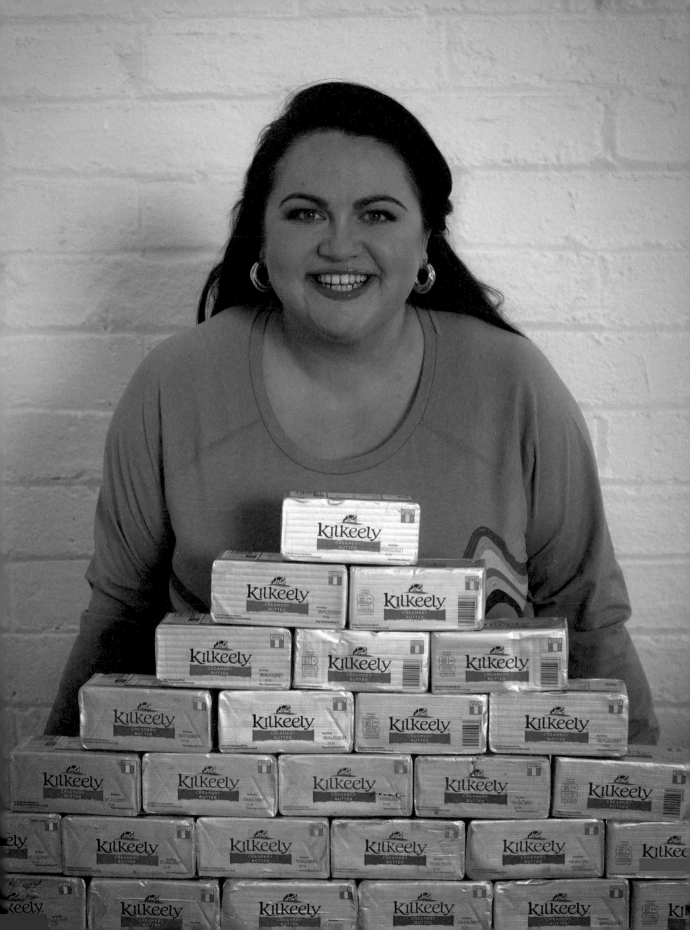

# HOW DO I RESET?

Now that you've answered the question that will form the basis for your reset plan, it's time to look at what you can do to reset. Here are the steps:

1 **Set a long-term goal.** What is your dream? For example, I want to lose seven stone in the next few years.

.......................................................................................................................

2 **Now break that long-term goal into a few small goals so it's not as daunting.** Three weeks is not a long time – anyone can manage three weeks, but the progress you can make in just 21 days should not be underestimated. Don't make any drastic moves like cutting out everything you love and don't make any blanket statements like 'I will never eat a chip again!' You are only setting yourself up for failure by doing that. I will break my long-term goal to lose seven stone into a smaller goal to lose one stone by the end of the year.

.......................................................................................................................

.......................................................................................................................

.......................................................................................................................

.......................................................................................................................

.......................................................................................................................

3  **Write a list of how you can achieve each of your smaller goals,** for example go to the gym three times a week, drink 2 litres of water every day, get at least 8 hours of sleep every night, go for a 30-minute walk three times a week, and batch-cook my dinners.

........................................................................................................

........................................................................................................

........................................................................................................

........................................................................................................

........................................................................................................

4  **Doing this alone makes it harder,** so write a list of who you can contact to help you achieve your goals. It doesn't matter who it is – it could be a family member for support, a Slimming World consultant, a personal trainer at a gym or a friend to go on walks with. You won't lose any extra pounds for doing this alone, so you might as well get someone to give you a hand.

........................................................................................................

........................................................................................................

........................................................................................................

........................................................................................................

5 **See where in your schedule you can dedicate some time to achieve all your goals.** Write down what you can do. Can you reduce your screen time? Can you bring your family on your walks? Can you slot in a time that doesn't change for your weekly shop? Planning is so important for the end result. You know what they say – if you fail to prepare, prepare to fail. Once you have a roadmap in front of you, it's easier and clearer for you to see the main objective, which is to feel good.

...................................................................................................

...................................................................................................

...................................................................................................

...................................................................................................

6 **Do a stock take of your cupboards and make a shopping list.** We waste so much money on buying new things. If you're anything like me, you end up with six jars of cumin in the press! It takes five minutes and is so satisfying when you know that you're saving money and calories by not buying the extra bits 'just in case.'

...................................................................................................

...................................................................................................

...................................................................................................

...................................................................................................

...................................................................................................

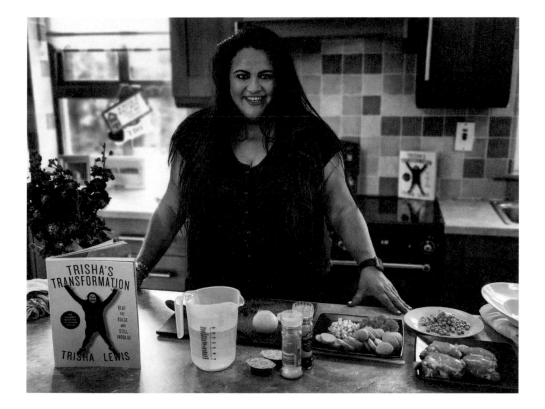

7 **Pick a day to start.** Don't feel under pressure to start on a Monday or the first day of the month or the start of a new year. This is your personal plan, so start when it feels right.

........................................................................................................................

8 **Smile!** You're about to start a new life, one that you have always dreamed of.

# HOW DO I STAY FOCUSED?

Oh lord above, if I had a euro for every time I wished for motivation, I would be a very wealthy woman! Wishing for motivation is like wishing for a unicorn to walk past you in a shopping centre. You can try, but it won't happen. I have spent so much money on the promise of motivation and now I feel like I spent it buying some magic beans. Motivation is fleeting, and in my opinion it doesn't even exist in the way that it's sold to us.

I think that the ability to reset over and over again is the motivation we all desire. Hear me out. The most motivated people in the world are just people who are resilient to failure and have the ability to reset over and over again. I stay focused because I know just how good my body should feel, so now when I feel sad or down I know that I have the power to apply some simple methods and get back on track. Staying focused is hard, but what makes it easier for me is knowing that setbacks are going to happen but that I can keep resetting and making sure I am adjusting my journey. Setting smart, realistic goals and taking it day by day is a game-changer.

**In order to stay focused and keep resetting, there are six key areas you need to embrace:**

- **Questions and curveballs**
- **Hard work**
- **Discipline**
- **Time management**
- **Courage**
- **Accountability**

## EMBRACE THE QUESTIONS AND CURVEBALLS

When I open my eyes each morning, I ask myself three questions before I take my head off the pillow: Do I want to be fat or fit? Happy or sad? Healthy or dying? And I go from there.

Curveballs will be thrown at you all day long and temptation will be lurking around every corner. Sometimes I make a rash decision about what to eat, but these next two questions have helped me so much to stay focused:

● **Do I want this now?** Usually the answer is yes.
● **Will this benefit me in one year's time and get me closer to my goal?** Usually the answer is absolutely not. (So put down that chocolate bar!)

These questions are an amazing tool to have in your toolbox. If you still decide to have the food you're being tempted by, at least you'll be aware of your decision, not just mindlessly eating. Like my 'why' questions, these two questions help me make day-to-day decisions.

## EMBRACE HARD WORK

There is no way to sugar-coat weight loss. It's hard work. You have to make a choice – either don't do it and have a hard day 24/7 or work hard for about one hour per day. For example, at the start of my weight loss journey I let myself off lightly with exercise, but in the end it was much harder than if I had just done it. The hard work isn't just the exercise, it's also changing your mindset. It's so rewarding looking back at what you have accomplished and knowing that it's all down to the decisions you make every day.

## EMBRACE DISCIPLINE

I think the hardest word to say in the English language is no, but for your weight loss journey to work, you have to learn how to say it during those times when motivation and willpower have abandoned you. Discipline is a verb – it's something that you do – whereas motivation is a noun, something that can come and go as it pleases. Self-discipline is tough, but like all habits, once it's done over and over again it becomes a natural reflex.

I think kids have it nailed. They eat intuitively and when they're full, they stop. End of. I love their discipline. We tend to overcomplicate this as adults.

When my nieces and nephews land up to the house I will pop on some food for them. It could be sausages, cereal or chicken, but I would often grab the last bit that they didn't have and mindlessly eat it. Later on I would say to myself, 'I haven't eaten anything bad today', but I had those two goujons. Add this up over the course of a year, and that's a serious amount of extra calories that you 'didn't' have.

Stop the random eating. If you pick one piece of chicken a day from your child's plate, that is 365 pieces of chicken a year that you're pretending you didn't have. Are you guilty of this? Call yourself out, Transformer. Kitchen pickers, bigger knickers!

**Working from home**
In all the years that I worked as a chef, I often thought that things would be so much easier if I worked from home and just had what I needed in the house. After changing my career a few months ago, I now do a lot of my work from the laptop at home and I've realised how wrong I was. For one thing, I'm not as physically active now. I also sometimes go through bouts of unproductivity, when I find myself randomly walking to the fridge and picking, so I had to set up boundaries and systems to prevent me from eating mindless calories. Working from home requires a lot more discipline around eating than I had originally thought!

Here is what I advise if you're struggling with working from home:

● **Get showered and dressed.** Put on a nice perfume or aftershave and some make-up to make yourself feel good. If you're sitting in your pyjamas with your hair all over the place, then you probably won't be bothered with your diet plan either. So spruce yourself up ... for you!

● **Work out first thing in the morning.** When you win your morning, it's easier to win the day. Use the time that you would have used on your commute. Instead of a moving car, move you!

● **Create a workspace.** Ideally, try not to work in the kitchen if at all possible. Separate your food from

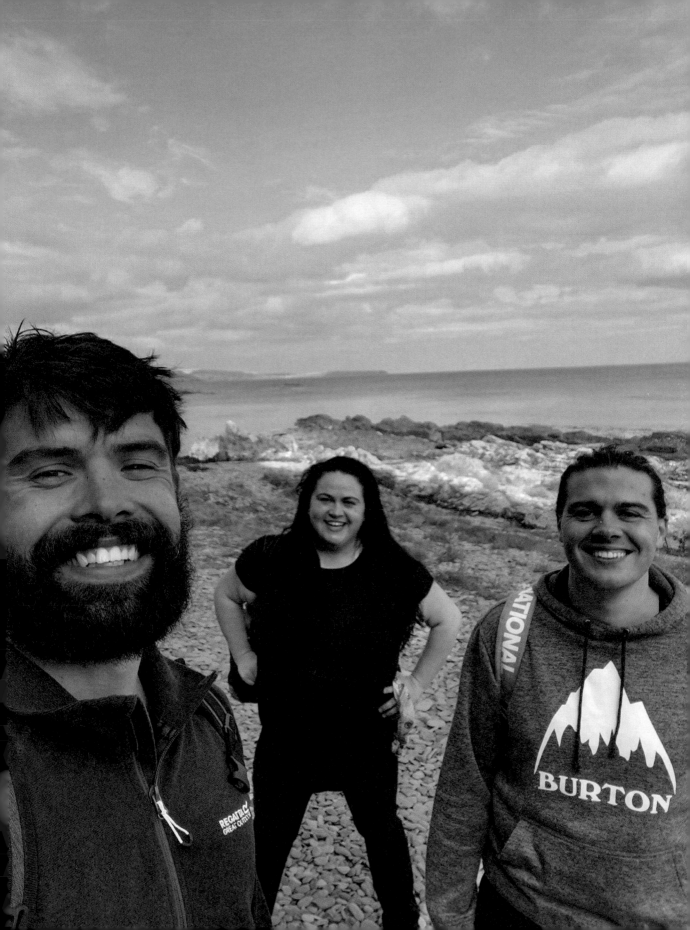

your work, otherwise you'll be wandering back and forth to the fridge like a puppy and convincing yourself that a random slice of cheese is what you want, and I promise you it isn't.

- **Plan your day.** Do this from the moment you get up and include the meals that you'll be having, then don't deviate from that. This is a boundary and a tool that is going to benefit you. You need to create discipline at home.

- **Make sure your meals are balanced.** If you're eating crap you'll feel like crap, so make sure you're getting plenty of protein and good fats from a balanced diet to keep you operating at your max.

- **Pack your lunch.** Pack your lunch in the morning like you would if you were working from an office, as you still need to take a lunch break even if you're working from home. When the weather is nice, go outside and eat your lunch in your garden.

- **Eat when you're meant to.** When we aren't in our regular environment it can sometimes be easier to just keep ploughing through work to finish your day earlier, but this

means you'll be too hungry by the end of the day and wind up overeating, which is obviously not a sustainable approach to weight loss. Eat when it's time to do so or when you're actually hungry.

- **Eat in a window.** I have a window of time that I eat in, as it helps me to have this boundary. I have breakfast at 10 a.m. and after 7 p.m. I don't eat another bite. Once 7:01 p.m. hits, the presses cannot be opened.

- **Don't use food as a way to pass some time.** Stock up on sparkling water and have a glass of that on ice with fresh lemon instead.

- **Set up a hydration station.** We often mistake thirst for hunger, so sip your water throughout the day. If you keep a bottle beside you, you increase your chances of hitting your water goal. When we are dehydrated it leads to fatigue, which leads to picking at food and hitting the self-sabotage button.

- **Don't buy multipacks.** This is vital. I know that if it's in the press it will be calling to me, and before I know it, I will have eaten my entire week's quota. To stop this, I had to stop buying! The hardest step in Aldi is

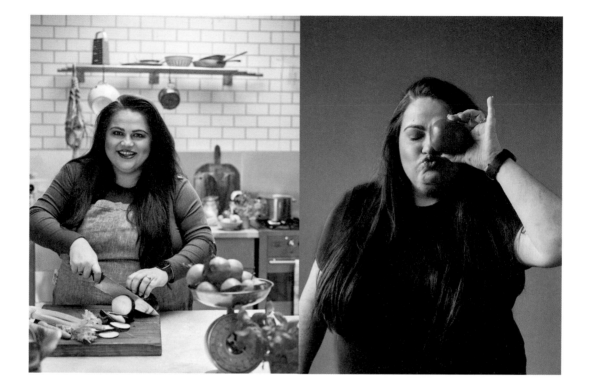

to not step down the sweet aisle, so save yourself the hassle and just skip it.

- **Call yourself out.** Leaning against the counter nibbling on some crackers or biscuits is never going to give you fulfilment or help you towards your end goal.

- **Batch cook.** Make extra portions of meals and prep ahead so that you never get so hungry that you just eat anything. This is especially true for lunch. Have some cooked chicken or spuds, washed lettuce, hummus and pepper slices on hand – whatever will help you to have a nice balanced lunch that you will look forward to.

- **Switch off.** When the clock strikes the time you finish work, stop checking your emails. It's exhausting being 'always on', and when you're overtired you will usually mindlessly eat or pick.

## EMBRACE TIME MANAGEMENT

This is vital. Manage your time, your actions and your choices. This can be simple things like prioritising your sleep or filling up your petrol tank if you're heading out on a long drive so that you aren't tempted by the sweets at the till.

- Don't go shopping hungry.
- Make a shopping list.
- Don't batch cook when you're hungry.
- Don't eat the remaining food from your kids' plates.
- Eat little and often to prevent hungry surges and binges.
- Manage your exercise – once it's written down, it must be done.

## EMBRACE COURAGE

This can be a hard one, as all too often we do things that we think will please or suit others. Have the courage to put yourself first in all scenarios. You have to be number one for everyone else to benefit. For example, when it comes to birthdays, parties or gatherings, if you don't want to drink, then don't. If you just want to have water at dinner, then do. In the long run, you have to have the courage to speak up and to make sure that every single move you make is as a Transformer.

## EMBRACE ACCOUNTABILITY

Accountability doesn't mean punish-ment – it means that you take responsibility for your actions, whether they are good or bad. It means that you accept who you are and want the best for yourself. But you can't only do this every so often. This needs to be a regular event for it to really work.

A lot of people ask me why I set up an Instagram page at 25 stone. The main reason was for accountability … to myself. For years I would go on a health kick and lose weight and I'd feel amazing, but then I would start enjoying myself more and becoming less disciplined. Before I knew it, I was back to feeling like crap, caught in the vicious circle of weight gain and feeling sad again.

Sometimes it can be hard to admit on Instagram when things go wrong and tell my Transformers that I am up weight or that I drank way too much, but lying about your struggles won't fix them, so make yourself accountable to someone. A lot of people use the scales as their sole accountability, but this is a recipe for disaster. Use the scales as a guide, but weight fluctuates sometimes, so don't attach too much emotion to them.

*If you were everyone's cup of tea, you would be a mug.*

The evening that I decided to set up my Instagram account, I remember sitting on the couch and my sisters and friends were giving me the pros and cons of what I was about to embark on. They were desperately worried that I would be mocked or trolled and that my mental health wouldn't be strong enough to handle it. I remember listening to them, but inside I knew that I had to do it for me. I know my own weaknesses and forgetting how crap I've felt is one of them, so I had to have this somewhere permanent.

When I set up that Instagram account, never in my wildest dreams did I think it would take off the way it has. I write from the heart because I want the future Trisha to know how tough it is to be overweight and sore. My captions are honest and true. Some might even be too much information, but what I need to explain is that those captions are for me and me alone. I set it up because I knew that at some point I would forget how it felt to be obese, which could make me go backwards. But once I had it all documented, I could always go back and reread what it felt like to not be able to shower or to buckle the seatbelt on a plane.

I can honestly say that setting up my Instagram page has been a huge part of my staying power on this journey, and as a Transformer I would urge you to do the same. If you feel like setting up your own page or telling your story is too much, then curate your feed to make sure the only things you see are tools that will help you in your journey. Follow pages that are true to you. Follow positive affirmations. Follow people who are also on a weight loss journey or who post good food. Every move you make, even what you consume on your phone, needs to be a stepping stone for you to get to your goal.

If you have a check-in and you know that your weight is up, remember that being up isn't a bad thing. Look at it as feedback that calories were consumed that could have been managed better, but don't fool yourself by dropping your accountability just because the answer isn't what you want it to be.

Think of the game, always. Think of the end goal. Sometimes being accountable can be hard because not every single week is going to be amazing, but you must stick with it through the good and the bad. Weight loss will never be linear, so what harm is there in having it documented? I look forward to seeing your Instagram pages. Use the word 'reset' in them and tag me so I can watch your progress! #resetwithtrisha

An Instagram page is just one way for you to be responsible for yourself and your health. Here are some other ways that you can have accountability:

- **Set up a WhatsApp group** and keep your friends updated.
- **Join Facebook groups** with likeminded people who ooze positivity.
- **Curate your social media feeds** to only show accounts that will help you reach your end goal.
- **Get a coach** or a personal trainer.
- **Use this planner,** get a biro and write everything down. It's so important for you to see what the goals and plan are on paper.

# HOW DO I LOVE MYSELF?

Self-care helps to form the foundation for resetting. It's the foundation for being able to embrace the curveballs, hard work, discipline, time management, courage and accountability.

On a physical level, this is something that I am only getting used to now. I never truly looked after myself because I never felt good enough. I always felt like it was too much work and that it's only what other girls do. For events like weddings, birthdays and christenings I would always wait until the day before to buy my dress. This was a form of self-sabotage because I didn't feel like I deserved to look or feel as good as everyone else.

For years I didn't comb my hair every day, I didn't shower every day and I didn't brush my teeth every day. Me time was always last on the agenda. I would prioritise Netflix and Instagram before I would think of brushing my hair or applying a face mask. It's embarrassing to admit, but I have always said I would tell the truth in every regard and this was the reality of not loving myself. My biggest downfall in self-care was my hygiene. I hated who I was, so I just didn't bother. When my hygiene slips, it's a huge indicator to me that I'm not on top of my game and looking after myself well.

If you are in the position that I used to be in, I urge you to change it, as it will make you feel so much better. Since I began my lifestyle journey, it has been such a lovely feeling looking after myself. Life is for living and a simple thing like starting your morning with a glass of water could change your whole day. Stop wearing the good clothes only on special occasions – wear that expensive top to the shop! – and use your nice perfume. Smelling good is so much nicer for you and everyone else.

## THERAPY HAS BEEN MY BEST INVESTMENT

But it's not just about looking after yourself on the outside. When we look after all aspects of our self, everything seems easier and much more manageable. But therapy was something that I always felt wasn't for me, that I wasn't 'that bad.' I am writing this down here because I want to let you know that therapy is one of the best investments I have ever made in myself in my life. I am an open person and I have family and friends I can talk to, but there is something different about therapy. There is no shame or stigma to it – it's the same thing as going to the doctor with a sore throat. A therapist can help you with a sore mind.

I go to therapy for an eating disorder called binge eating disorder (BED). Here is the definition of BED according to the Bodywhys website:

*Binge eating disorder (BED) is a recognised eating disorder in which a person, due to underlying issues and other risk factors, develops a pattern of binge eating which they come to rely on as a way of coping. In the same way as someone with anorexia and bulimia, the person with binge eating disorder feels compelled to continue with the disordered eating, i.e. binge eating, as a way of coping with emotional turmoil. It must be recognised that as with the other eating disorders, a person diagnosed with binge eating disorder cannot be treated by diet alone. All the eating disorders are serious mental disorders which require timely and appropriate treatment and support.*

For years I would eat food privately and eat so much that my stomach would hurt. I would want to lie down and go to sleep, repulsed at what I had done. I always felt like such a loser doing it and I would internally add another notch onto the self-hate ladder.

A few months ago I read some stuff about me online that was hurtful, but one of the lines that changed my life was, 'She needs to address that she has some sort of binge eating disorder.' When something hurts you, you have to look inside yourself to see why. I knew that it stung because I did have a problem.

# IF YOU ARE NOT CHANGING IT, YOU ARE CHOOSING IT

A few days later, I did some searching online and found my therapist. Sitting in front of my therapist for the first time, I was feeling quite down and upset. How could Trisha from Trisha's Transformation still be struggling? What I have learned over the last few months has been truly life changing. I always knew that I was an emotional eater, but I didn't know how to stop it. The reason I didn't know how to stop it was because I didn't have the tools that I have now.

Treating the symptom is amazing, but finding the cause is glorious.

My biggest personal downfall is loneliness. I have a huge family, the best friends in the world and the thousands of amazing Transformers who follow me on Instagram, but some days my heart is sore and I feel like the most alone human in the world. I couldn't figure it out. I was always at my worst on days off, after special occasions or when I was on my own in a restaurant or my car. Why did I mainly crumble during those times?

My therapist explained why this was happening and told me that every single person on this planet feels lonely, so in a weird way it made me feel better. I grew up in a large family of eight sisters and my mam and dad and I worked as a chef for 13 years in a career that was based around teamwork. Someone has always had my back. I have never grown to love my own company, so when I'm alone or after a big family event, I find it hard to cope and turn to emotional eating.

*Do not be embarrassed of your failures, learn from them and reset.*

Once it was explained to me, the relief that I felt was magical. Knowledge is power. Knowledge is a weapon that your inner demons do not like. I cannot stress enough the importance of talking to someone. I cannot express how vital I have found therapy to be. Everyone deserves the chance to talk to someone.

As part of my care plan, I have started to change in ways I never thought I could. When I feel lonely now, I'm able for it. I can deal with it and I can sit with it knowing that it will pass and that everyone else feels like this sometimes too.

I think saying that you're lonely has an air of taboo to it, like you're weird and no one wants to be your friend, but it's not. Open up, speak out. The year 2020 forced a lot of us away from family and friends, and loneliness is dangerous if it's left to fester. I am so much better now at picking up my phone and texting someone for a chat or asking to meet for a coffee, a walk or just a simple hello.

But your phone can make you feel alone too, so please bear that in mind. You can spend hours aimlessly watching other people's lives and in turn feeling empty. Stop scrolling through social media and have a real conversation with someone instead. My top tips here are:

- **Talk to someone professional.** Don't worry one bit – no one will judge you.
- **Talk to your family and friends.** Be honest. Explain that these feelings happen and that you're just putting it out there.
- **Put away your phone and reduce your screen time.** Live in the moment, don't live in an app.
- **Set boundaries, whether it's around your time, people or your space.** In the past I had no boundaries at all, and in the end I started to feel burned out. Always remember that you can't give from an empty cup. My main boundary now is that I keep my therapy private. It may seem selfish, but I know that one of my downfalls is that I'm a people pleaser. Therapy has helped me identify so much about myself and I'm so grateful for it.

- **Be present.** As I type this, I have my phone on airplane mode because otherwise I would be mindlessly picking it up. I do the same when I'm in a room with people – I have to remind myself to take my head out of the phone.
- **Go for a 10-minute walk with no technology** – 5 minutes from your front door and 5 minutes back – and just absorb the sounds, the air and the colours.

When you are searching for a therapist, here are some things you should look out for:

- **Check reviews** online if possible.
- **Reach out** to places for advice that specialise in your area of concern.
- **Make sure** the therapist is accredited.
- **Give the therapist a chance**, but if you feel like it isn't working, find someone else. Sometimes it takes time to click and sometimes it just won't work – I'm on my second attempt at therapy. Never settle if your gut is off. This is too important.

*Am I cured? No. Therapy has taught me how to manage the BED and loneliness and that is like winning the lotto.*

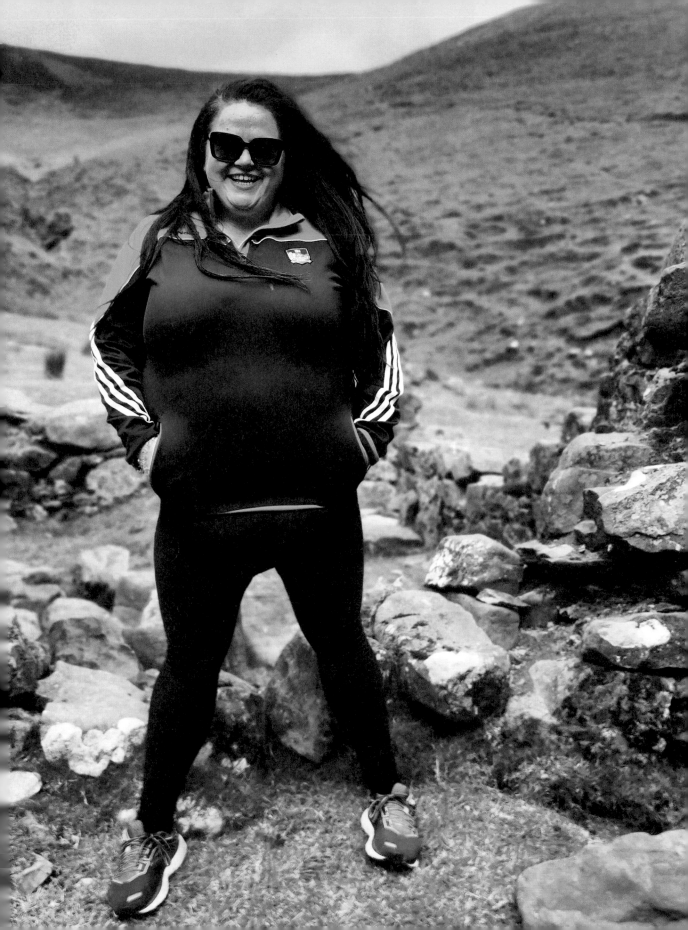

## THE CONTRACT

My therapist asked me to create a contract with myself. These are things that truly make me feel good and happy. When I start to struggle, she wants me to look at the contract to see if I am achieving everything that I should be, and if I'm not, it's a key indicator that things are going wrong.

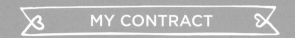

## MY CONTRACT

- ☐ Shower.

- ☐ Brush my teeth.

- ☐ Read 10 pages of my book.

- ☐ Eat four to five small meals per day.

- ☐ Drink a minimum of 2 litres of water.

- ☐ Leave my phone in the kitchen when I'm going to sleep. (Buy an alarm clock instead of using the alarm on your phone – no excuses!)

- ☐ Drink a cup of coffee in the morning and no coffee after 2 p.m.

- ☐ Get fresh air with a walk that is at least 15 minutes.

- ☐ Chat with Mam.

- ☐ Keep my screen time to under five hours.

In the box below, create your own contract. Keep it simple. Make sure they are things you can do every day.

## YOUR CONTRACT

1. ................................................................................................

2. ................................................................................................

3. ................................................................................................

4. ................................................................................................

5. ................................................................................................

6. ................................................................................................

7. ................................................................................................

8. ................................................................................................

9. ................................................................................................

10. ...............................................................................................

Signed ................................................ Date ................................

## NEGATIVE AND UNSUPPORTIVE PEOPLE

When you start changing your life and becoming happier, it's been my experience that negative people will not like it. These people can be someone close to you, someone you work with or someone on the internet.

The inner circle that you hold close will be another vital key in your journey. Your family and friends might be tired of hearing about every diet plan that you go on, so if they don't seem interested this time, do me a favour and smile to yourself because this is it – this is the moment you will show them that you are resetting for good! The first 50 times I started a new plan I gave up except for this time, so don't worry. The people who matter will eventually see what you are at.

Negative people are always going to be around. People who don't understand weight will always be around. They aren't your issue. You can't sort that out, but you can control the controllable here. Negative energy is so bad to have in your zone. The less you respond to negative people, the more peaceful your life will become. Always remember that at first they may laugh, but afterwards they will ask you how you did it.

I know this sounds ironic coming from someone with an Instagram page with thousands of followers, but keep your world small. If your world and your inner circle are diluted with too many people who may have too many opinions, you might struggle. You need everyone to support you on this journey, so if someone scoffs at you, encourages you to eat poorly or just doesn't seem to want it for you, then you have to put yourself first.

*Don't listen to criticism from someone you wouldn't take advice from.*

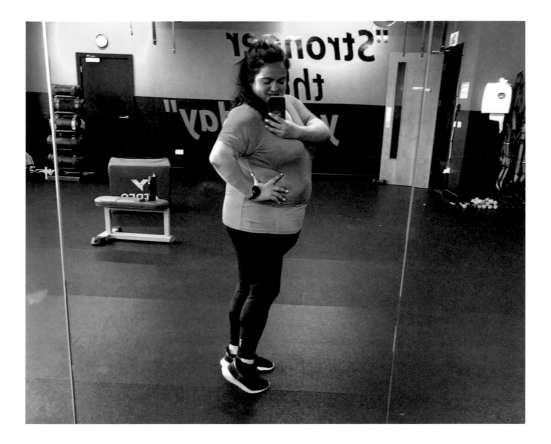

If you feel bad after leaving a coffee date, guilty for being happy or nervous that they won't give you praise or encouragement, then you may have to look at the following points:

1.  **Eliminate the person from your life completely** if they are truly toxic.
2.  **Limit time spent with negative people if you can't eliminate them.** It's easy to simply say, 'No, I'm going for a walk.' That's it. Don't overthink it – you are putting yourself first.
3.  **Set boundaries.** If people walk all over you and you are a classic people pleaser, like me, then start setting some boundaries. Don't be always available.

In every fairy-tale there is always a hero, and that hero is you. You are the hero in your fairy-tale but it's no harm having a few cheerleaders cheering you on!

# HOW TO HELP SOMEONE WHO MAY BE STRUGGLING WITH THEIR WEIGHT

Over the years my weight has been mentioned to me both kindly and cruelly, and strangely, both of them hurt in different ways. I am writing this for two people: the person who is worried about someone else's weight and the person who is carrying the weight. It's awkward for the person saying it and it's awkward for the person hearing it. It isn't easy to say it or to hear it. I understand that.

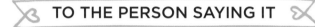

## TO THE PERSON SAYING IT

Before speaking to someone you're worried about, I have the following tips to give you. But most of all, trust me when I say this: BE POSITIVE. I am so blessed with my sisters and friends because I know they all believe in my ability to beat the bulge. When I stumble, they never focus on the setback. They always remind me of my accomplishments and encourage me to pick myself back up and move on.

- **Make sure it's your place to say it.** It isn't your place if you aren't going to follow it up with a support plan.

- **Have a second move planned.** If you're going to say it, then expect a reaction and accept that it may not be the one that you were hoping for. It could be aggressive or upsetting, but don't take it personally.

- **Do it gently and be kind.** No matter how awkward it is for you, it's 10 times worse for the other person.

- **Encourage them to adopt a healthier lifestyle** instead of using the words fat or weight loss.

- **Don't say it when they're eating.** I used to feel like such a waste of space when I was eating and someone would mention it to me.

- **Don't text it.** Do it face to face, as it's more empathetic that way.

- **Give some options of what they can do.** Check out the examples of my list of actionable goals on page 62: join a gym, drink lots of water, follow a meal plan, get enough sleep.

- **Reassure them that you love them** and that you just want them to be happier and healthier.

- **Offer to meet up for walks and chats.** Become an active person in their new lifestyle.

- **Be supportive.** Don't scoff a take-away in front of the person and then

# IF YOUR DREAMS DO NOT SCARE YOU, THEY ARE NOT BIG ENOUGH

expect them to eat a salad. Make sure you're doing your very best to implement healthy choices.

- **Be the cheerleader, not the trainer.** Don't pick at mistakes that the person may be making with their diet and lifestyle. At all times, praise and encourage the success as well as the flaws.
- **Make sure they know that you care about them, not the diet.** The diet is just a side effect of a healthier friend.
- **When they have a bad day, listen and do not judge.** Just tell them they are amazing and that tomorrow you will reset together.

- **Be aggressively supportive.** Make sure you always tell them that you are there for them. Get invested in each step they take and be so invested that they can't help but be excited too.
- **Find non-food ways to celebrate losses:** walks, random sea swims, a trip to the cinema or go-karting! Make it a good memory.
- **Don't take it personally if the first time doesn't work.** As the saying goes, you can bring a horse to water but you can't make it drink. So just regroup and try again another time.

## TO THE PERSON HEARING IT

- **The truth hurts,** but it might be what you needed to hear.
- **Have compassion for the other person.** This is coming from a place of love and care for you.
- **Know that you are enough** and that the reason this person is saying this is because if you didn't turn up in the morning, they would be heartbroken.
- **See this as a positive** and as the first step.
- **Prove the haters wrong.** If someone fat shames you, let them off but retaliate by proving them wrong. They will never expect your next move, which is to finally give yourself the chance to be happy.
- **Always remember that a thousand people could tell you this, but you are the one with the power.** Remember: if it is to be, it is up to me!

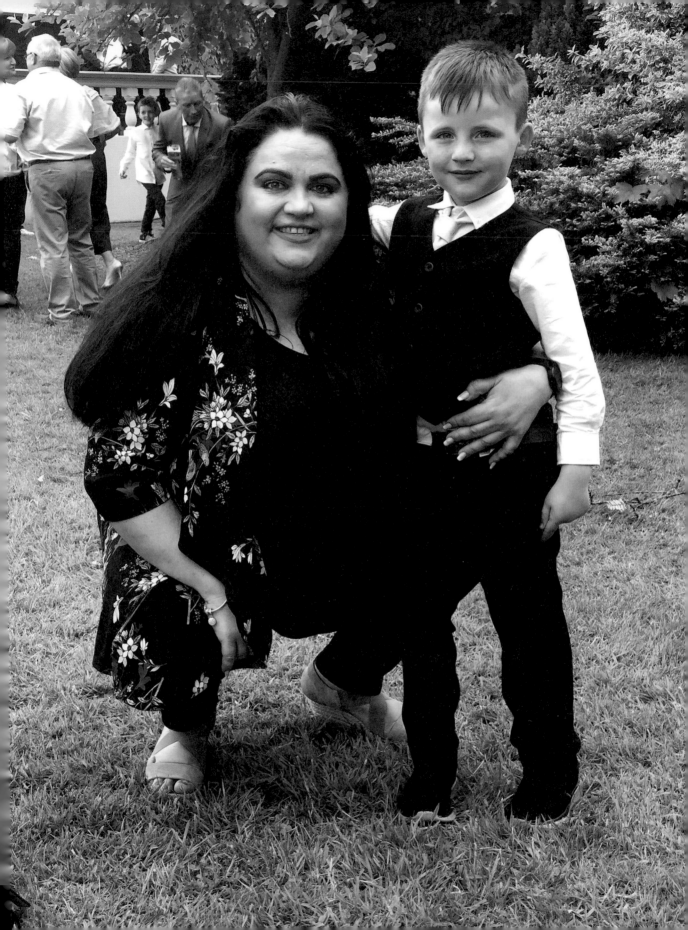

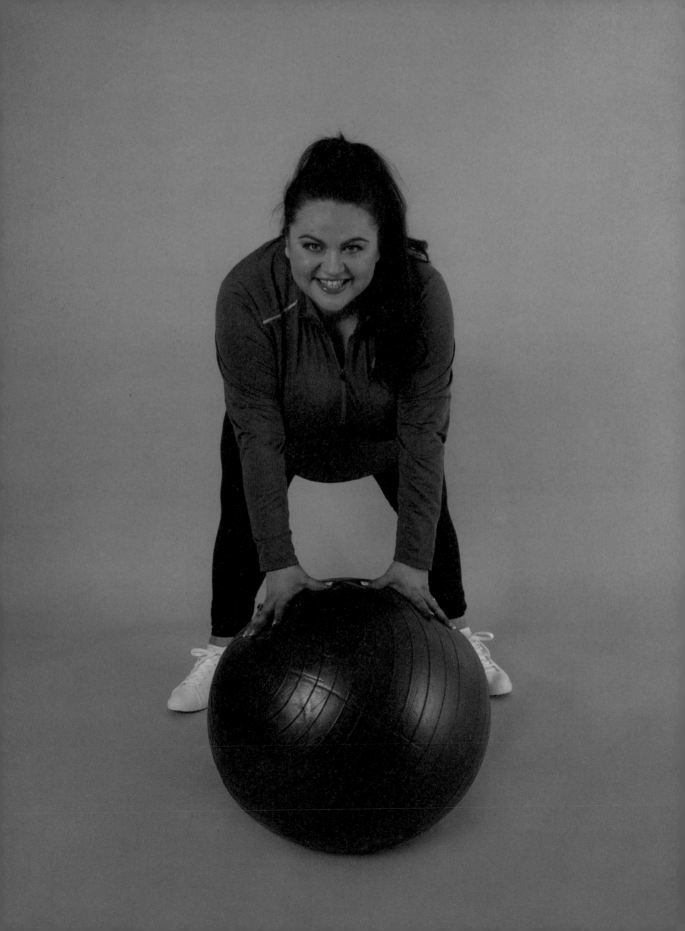

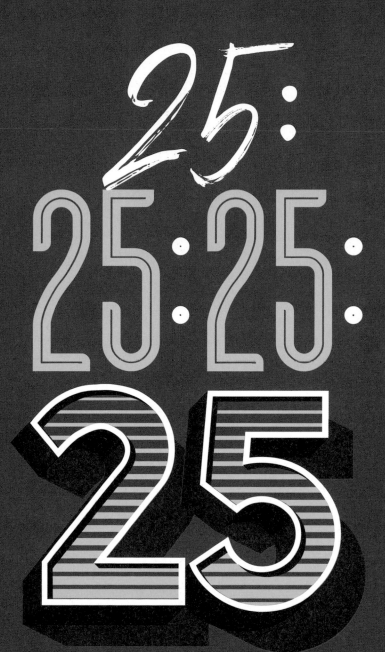

During the second lockdown in 2020, I was chatting to my sisters Annie, Carol and Maura. I was upset and struggling, as I felt like I was losing my way on my weight loss journey. I was bored and lonely and the nights were painfully long. In all my life as a chef, I never knew that the evenings were so long in the winter – I spent years in kitchens with no windows, so it had never bothered me before!

So anyway, I decided to start my 21-day reset. I was out on my third walk of the week and it felt like the fog was slowly lifting. I was starting to feel confident that I had control again and I was managing better. I was thinking about the 21 days and wondering why it felt so doable, and I realised it's the number that appeals to me. Then it clicked for me. The main reset I focus on is four factors to make sure that I feel 100%: water, exercise, sleep and nutrition. And just like that, 25:25:25:25 was born. I think I heard the 80:20 rule every single time I started a new diet and I just never clicked with it. The gist of the rule is that weight loss is 80 per cent the food you eat and 20 per cent exercise, but it doesn't work for me because it's missing two factors that I really need: sleep and water. I find that if I am missing those two, I can eat well and walk all I want, but I still feel like crap.

If you're struggling, look at each of these four areas and see which one you're not giving a full 25% to. You will see that all four factors play a harmonious tune together, and when all of these are being achieved, you are well and truly on the way to the grand reset.

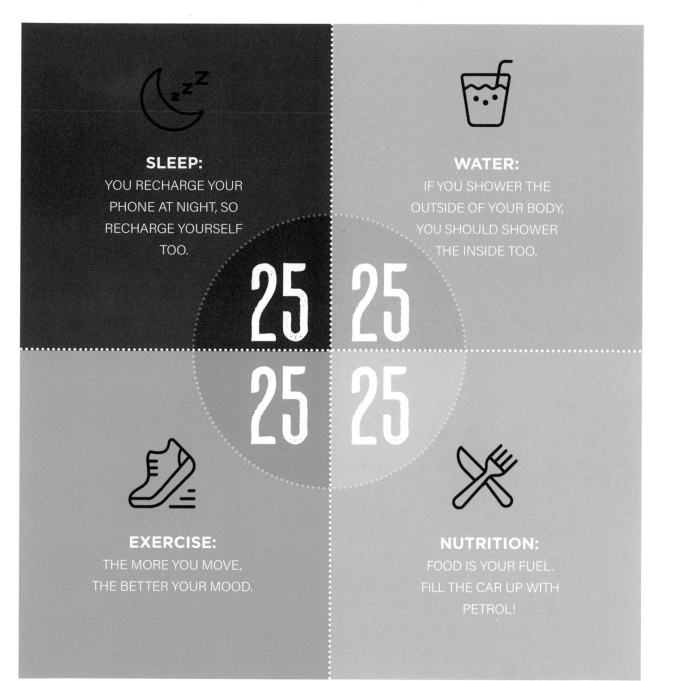

**SLEEP:**
YOU RECHARGE YOUR PHONE AT NIGHT, SO RECHARGE YOURSELF TOO.

**WATER:**
IF YOU SHOWER THE OUTSIDE OF YOUR BODY, YOU SHOULD SHOWER THE INSIDE TOO.

25  25

25  25

**EXERCISE:**
THE MORE YOU MOVE, THE BETTER YOUR MOOD.

**NUTRITION:**
FOOD IS YOUR FUEL. FILL THE CAR UP WITH PETROL!

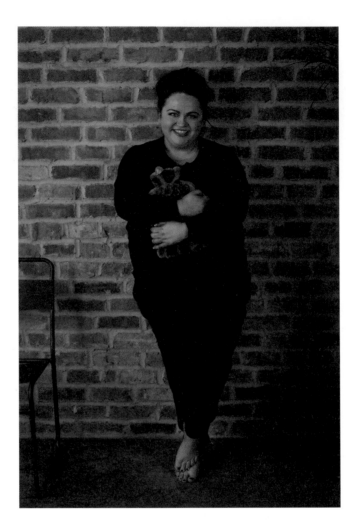

# 25: Sleep

I didn't get a full night's sleep for years. I would often dream (pardon the pun!) of what it would be like to go to sleep at 11 p.m. and wake up at 7 a.m., uninterrupted. I spent every night waking on the hour, every hour. I lost so many hours of sleep because of stress and worry. I was terrified that Mam would find me dead in the morning and I was always so stressed that someone would walk into my room and see my stomach if it was hanging out. I used to lie in my bed at night and get so upset at how crap my life was. I never thought I would see the day when I would sleep practically straight through.

Sleep is vital to your health. Like all other parts of your journey, this has to be prioritised. If I don't have a good sleep, I'm more prone to pick at food the next day and I don't push myself to my potential. When we sleep, our body recovers from the day and makes us feel refreshed. When I have a poor night's sleep, I find that the next day I'm much hungrier and I definitely have less control.

Rest is recovery and it will help you in your weight loss journey. Lack of good-quality sleep makes your fat cells sluggish, moody and grumpy, so they won't budge as quickly as they should. So if you aren't sleeping as well as you should be and would like to change this, here is what I did.

- **I removed my smartwatch and stopped checking how much I slept.** All that data wasn't much good to me when I was wrecked.
- **I removed my phone from my bedroom.** This was awful – I missed it so much! When I would wake at night searching for my phone like a child searching for a soother, it really proved to me how addicted I was.
- **I got an eye mask to block out any light.** I got a nice thick one, as I found thin straps were brutal and would fall off.
- **I started to take magnesium.** This is a game changer! It helps you sleep and it also relaxes your muscles. I take the MAG365 supplement. (Check out my Instagram Story highlights for more information!)
- **I started a routine of going to bed at the same time every night** so that my body started to get tired when it was supposed to.
- **I stopped drinking coffee after 2 p.m.,** which is eight hours before my bedtime.

All of these take effort, but they work. Turn off Netflix and go to sleep. Retrain yourself back to what bedtime was like when you were a child and you simply went to bed and went to sleep. I now go to sleep easily and when I wake I usually get up straight away – mainly because my phone is in the kitchen and I want to go on it!

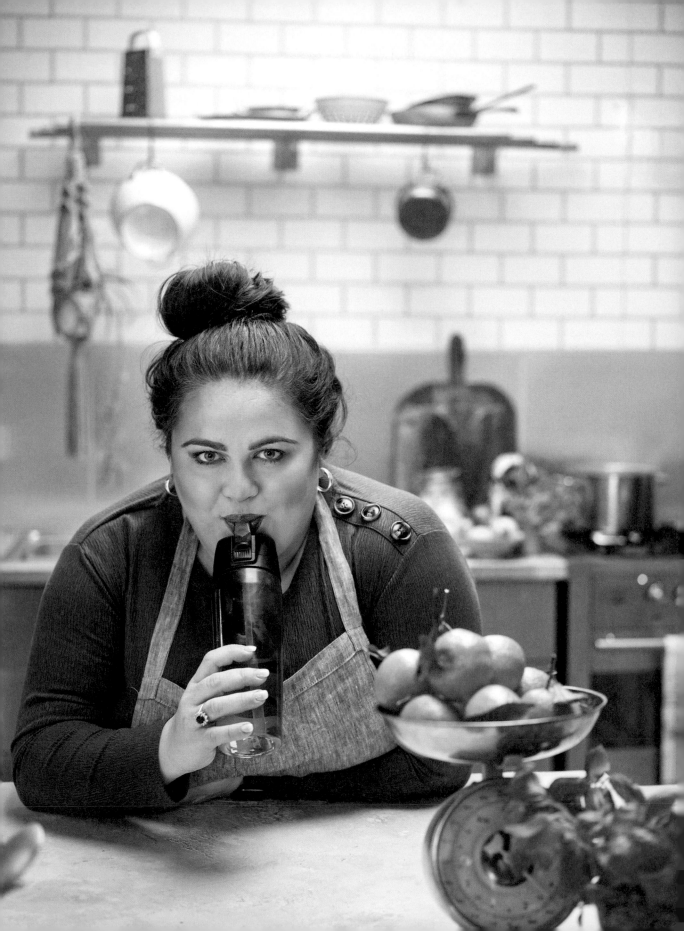

# 25: Water

Hell no, H$_2$O? Well, that should be a hell yes!

I know that at the start of a lifestyle change, one of the worst things is the constant need to go to the bathroom because you are drinking so much water. And think of it as a choice between drinking loads of water, feeling better and having to go to the loo every hour or not drinking water, feeling sluggish and not peeing every hour. And look on the bright side – you're getting your steps up walking back and forth from the toilet. At the start of my journey I spent more money on water bottles than anything else, as I kept leaving them all over Cork city. The bottles became an extension of my hand!

It's very easy to drop the ball on this one, as it can be monotonous to always be drinking water, but like all things in your lifestyle change, you must make this into a habit. Once it becomes a habit and you implement the discipline and give yourself no choice, soon enough you will end up craving it and it will be no bother to you. Now when I'm struggling with my water intake, especially in the winter, when it's harder to consume as much I like, I remind myself that my body is made up of 60–70% water and I think of Sandra Bullock in the movie *Speed*, where the dial can't go below a certain number, otherwise I'll blow up!

Water plays a huge part in feeling good and healthy. A key sign for me that I haven't drunk enough water in a day is puffy eyes and swollen fingers. When you are dehydrated you will be swollen and bloated, as your body can't remove excess waste efficiently and this will slow down your digestion. I find that when I'm drinking lots of water, my skin is clear and hydrated, my hair is glossy and I have a lot more energy. I'm also less likely to hit the 3 p.m. slump when I'm drinking the correct amount of water. Life is just easier when I'm hydrated.

I have also learned that I can often misread hunger when it's actually thirst. If I have eaten my meals but am craving a snack, I'll have a glass of water first and that satisfies me if it was thirst. Water is calorie free and this alone is a huge bonus to changing your lifestyle.

I often get asked how to kick a mineral or soft drink addiction. My answer is to reduce, not remove. If you're making a lifestyle change and remove every single thing you enjoy, it will not be sustainable. If, for example, you drink 10 cans of full-sugar Coke per day and reduce that to zero, you will be miserable and are only setting yourself up to fail. Instead, I suggest switching to sugar-free soft drinks and reducing your consumption by half. Replace what you have removed with water instead. Slowly change your habits so eventually you will reach for a bottle of water over a bottle of sugar.

Water is so important when you are looking to change your lifestyle and the benefits outweigh the constant urge to pee. Your goal must be attainable for this to work, so here are my top tips on how to keep hydrated.

- **Set a realistic consumption goal and get that habit formed.** Start with 1 litre, then increase that by 100ml each week. Progress slowly and surely.
- **Use a sugar-free dilute or fresh fruit** (try strawberry and mint, lemon and cucumber, or orange and raspberry) to flavour your water, which can help you to drink more of it.
- **Chill your water.** I find that it's much nicer this way.
- **Get a good water bottle.** I prefer the ones with straws, as they are easier to drink from. I may sound precious, but I have to have a good water bottle. I see it as an investment to not buy bigger clothes in the future.
- **Know the volume of your water bottle so that you know where you are at.** For example, my bottle holds 625ml, so I aim to drink four bottles a day for a total of 2.5 litres.
- **Sip all day as opposed to slugging back a few litres.** Try setting an alarm on your phone to drink a certain amount of water every 30 minutes.

- **I always drive with a bottle of water beside me in the cup holder** so it stops me craving a snack while driving.
- **Record your progress in your phone or diary and take pictures of your skin each day.** Compare the before-and-after pictures after a month to see the difference!
- **Add a spicy meal to your plan** – this is a sure way of getting water into you!
- **Stop drinking water about 3 hours before your bedtime** (but start drinking it the minute you wake up), as if you're drinking too much too late, your sleep will be interrupted by getting up for the loo! Get the balance right so that your water factor isn't negatively affecting your sleep factor.
- **Remember that if you shower the outside of your body,** you must also shower the inside of your body!

Don't give yourself a choice on this one. Drinking water is essential on your trek to a healthier lifestyle. Don't say you hate water – you literally have to suck it up!

*Life has offered you a second chance. It is called today.*

# 25: Exercise

## I've been there

Exercise has been such a huge part of my journey, but I'll be honest – for years I dreaded the gym, walking, running, Zumba or anything that involved my heart rate going through the roof. I was so embarrassed by how unfit I was that I just didn't start. In hindsight, my heavy breathing and burning chest were just feedback that I needed to mind my body more, not something to be ashamed of.

So many times over the years, I would read some amazing testimonial on Facebook or Instagram and I would message the gym or person straight away and ask how it could be done. But once the reply came in, I didn't respond. That was it. I had asked the question with no real intention of starting. At the time I thought I was lazy and I would be so mad at myself, but the truth was I had no other plan made, only to contact the person. This is so hard on your head, as you will count this as another failure when it's not – you're only human. I remember never starting because I felt it was going to be too hard. The truth is, once I started and I committed to exercising three times a week for 30 minutes, it became my life and it was nowhere near as bad as I thought it was going to be.

I'm not here to lie to you and tell you this was the easiest habit I've ever picked up. It was awful at the start. I was so disgusted at myself because I wore black pyjama bottoms for the first few weeks, as that is all that would fit me. The underside of my stomach was inflamed with sores and it was red and raw from all the extra movement. I cried more often than not leaving the gym because all I felt was fatness. I didn't see what I see now. I didn't see just how bloody strong I was. I didn't see people looking at me with admiration. But I see now how brave I was, how wonderful it was to see a 26-stone woman in the gym. This does change. I don't know when, but I guess it's like the new kid in school – eventually you feel like they've always been there. That's what happened to me, anyway. It was amazing when I realised that once I managed my food and water intake better, I began to actually enjoy the workouts.

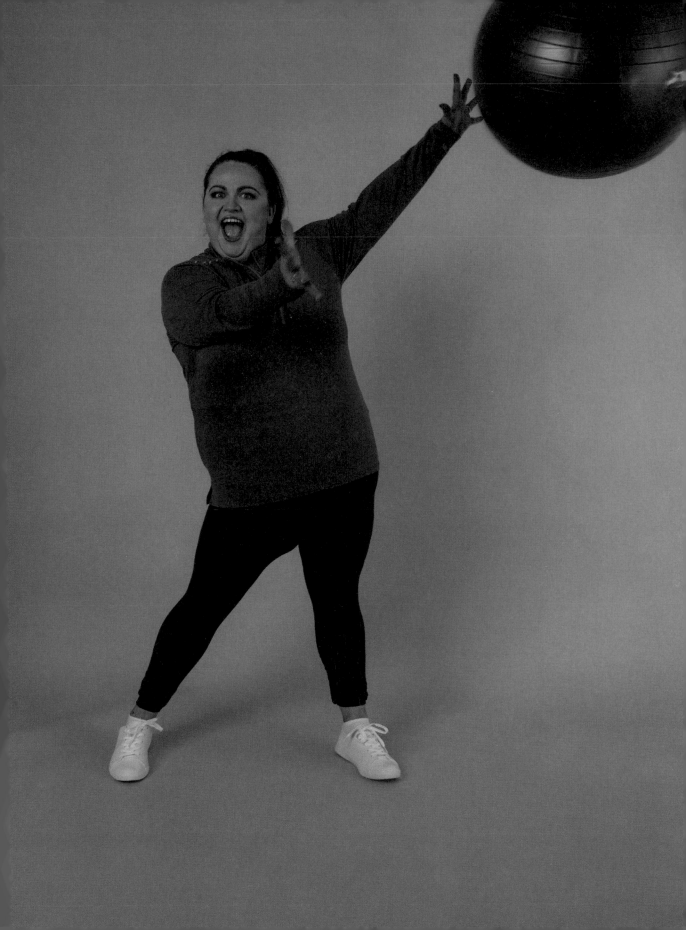

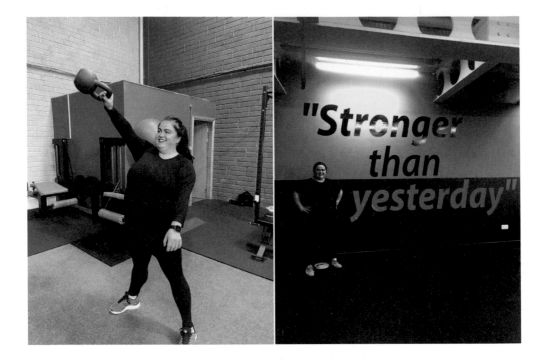

Exercise was always something someone else did. It was never something I did. I struggled to walk, never mind work out. If I had to go up a flight of stairs, I would try to think of a way to get someone else to go up for me. I would get dizzy picking up a biro. One night when I was on holiday in Marbella with friends, there was a taxi strike and we had to walk home. I spent an hour on the curb calling taxi numbers over and over again. I felt so helpless, as I couldn't tell the girls what was wrong and no one was answering my calls. When we eventually started walking home, I kept convincing the girls to stop for a cigarette and chats just so I could ease the pain I was in. My knees were in bits and the underside of my belly was bleeding from the chafing and the heat.

After some time, a cab drove past and I flagged him down. I begged the driver to bring me home. Eventually we came to an agreement that I would pay him €50 to drop me the 2km home and my friend Laura hopped in with me. She hadn't witnessed our chat, so when we pulled up outside the apartment and I paid the man €50 and hopped out, Laura was like, hold tough and get your change. I remember how horrified she was, as she thought we'd been robbed, but the truth was I couldn't walk. We never mentioned it again until recently, when we were having coffee with Shelly, who had also been on that holiday with us. That holiday in Marbella was the first time I didn't go to the beach, as there was an uphill incline home and I knew I wouldn't be able for it. I can't wait to return with Shelly and Laura and skip down to the beach with them and really enjoy my holiday with two of my favourite people in the world.

The reason I'm telling you this story is because I know what it's like. I know how scared you are and how you feel like you're going to collapse with exhaustion at any minute. That no one on this planet is as unfit as you are. I know what it's like to be walking down the street, roasting and out of breath, your heart heavy with shame. I know what it's like as people run their eyes down and stare at your stomach. I know what it's like to see people nudge each other as you approach.

I am telling you that you can change this. I now know what it's like to run up stairs without thinking, to hurry down the street without feeling like I'll collapse on the ground. People still stare and nudge each other if I am in brightly coloured leggings, but I'm proud now of who I am, so it doesn't affect me as much anymore.

Exercise freed me from a life sentence in prison. Each day that I exercise, I feel like I'm adding another day onto my life. Each time I'm uncomfortable sweating for 30 or 45 minutes, I know that I'm making the remaining 23-hours-and-a-bit of the day more enjoyable. The truth is that exercise is for every single one of us. We were born to move. You will not get the ass you want by sitting on the ass you have!

I was that girl who walked into the gym with a torn cardigan, unwashed hair and feeling like the biggest loser in the world. I now know what it feels like to not have a care in the world. So stop standing in your own way!

## NAME YOUR FEARS AND ADDRESS THEM HEAD ON

I think we all have nightmares of PE in school, having to work out in the school tracksuit and not being as fast as the sporty person. Get rid of that fear and take back control. Stand up to your inner bully telling you that you can't do this. Bullies are cowards and immediately become smaller when challenged. Do any of these unhelpful thoughts sound familiar?

**'You will be laughed at.'**

**'You won't be able.'**

**'You will be judged.'**

**'You will give up.'**

**'You will die of a heart attack.'**

**'You don't even know where to start.'**

**'You will have excess skin.'**

I get all of this. Let me assure you these are all real concerns, but your inner bully is feeding you with self-doubt and lies. They aren't going to stop you. You are reading this book and you have hope. You know you can do it and I know you can too.

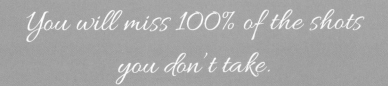

*You will miss 100% of the shots you don't take.*

## BUILD A RELATIONSHIP WITH A PERSONAL TRAINER

No one cares how you look in the gym. They are there for themselves, just like you are. You might worry that a trainer will judge you for not knowing how to squat, but that's like a baker judging you for not knowing how to make brioche. It's irrational. You may have been to a trainer, class or gym in the past and are embarrassed to go back. Trust me when I say that this doesn't matter. At the end of the day, they are doing their job and their job is to not judge. Your worry is unnecessary. The quicker that you get over these fears, the quicker you will become a Transformer.

Finding a personal trainer is all about building up trust, communication and fun. This won't happen for a little while. The first few sessions are just as awkward for the personal trainer as it is for you, as they need to get to know you too. You have to tell them the truth. No more secret eating and no more blame. Always tell the trainer the truth, the whole truth and nothing but the truth. If you have had a bad week, tell them and don't blame your metabolism like I did! The more they know, the easier the task at hand becomes.

When you are looking for a personal trainer, check that their testimonials are real and that there are at least a few of them. Ask them if they've ever trained someone your size. Make sure the session is about you and that you have their attention. Open up a line of communication.

This all might feel awful but it's not your trainer's fault, so don't not go back. Go back every day and get it done. This will require discipline and consistency. Be realistic. At 27 stone I knew that I needed help, so I went for personal training because if I hadn't done it by myself by that stage, I knew that I never would.

Being fat and going to the gym is usually tied into a negative. It's like a punishment for gaining weight. We think it should be awful and hard and you shouldn't love it while you're doing it. I felt that way for years, but then one day I realised that I had the power to flip that attitude. I stopped seeing myself as a fat person and started calling myself an athlete. The way I see it, an athlete does their very best with the body and power that they have at that moment in time, so I decided that was me. This was a huge turning point in my journey. I stopped seeing exercise as punishment and started realising that I was giving myself a gift every single time I lunged, squatted and jumped. Don't get me wrong, some days I want to fire the kettlebell at my trainers, Emma or Niall, but it's all part of the fun.

## LEAVE YOUR EGO AT THE DOOR

What did I do differently this time than all the other times? I left my ego at the door. I listened. I stopped thinking I knew how to squat and I started from scratch. I let the professional (Emma) do her job and I communicated. I told her when weights could go up and I told her when I was having a bad day. I stopped overcompensating and chatting to distract people from my weight. I let the tears fall when I was embarrassed and I let my smile shine when I was happy. I let go.

I also did something that I hadn't ever done before: I took pride in my work and I stopped speaking badly to myself in my head. I stopped calling myself fat as I struggled with my range of motion. I told myself to relax and that, yes, it was hard now, but I would get there. Rome wasn't built in a day. I guided myself internally through each session and every single day I told myself that I was proud of myself, even when sometimes I didn't believe it.

I had spent so many years making fun of myself and being ashamed of my size that I often didn't speak up, so when I was put on a treadmill for too long and got bored, I would just leave the gym. This isn't a smart move. Communication is key here. If you need to slow things down or shake things up, do! There's nothing wrong with that. If you're being lazy, that's a different story. Make sure you can identify when you are because you need to nip it!

# GROWTH BEGINS WHEN WE START TO ACCEPT OUR WEAKNESSES

## THE GYM IS NOT FOR EVERYONE

Now I know that the gym is not for everyone's personal budget or taste and that's okay, but you can't let that deter you from changing your life. You don't need all the gadgets in the world. You don't need a fitness watch and seven different gym outfits. Buy a pair of good runners and go walking. I swear by investing in good shoes to make sure you are preventing injury as much as you possibly can. I will always go to an expert (Mark and the gang at John Buckley Sports in Cork know what they are talking about). If you are starting from scratch, please don't go walk 10k or start running. Start with a walk with no hills and go for 10 minutes four times a week. Slowly increase the time when your walking pushes you so that you are slightly out of breath and your blood is pumping. Stop giving yourself excuses and start giving yourself reasons to smile.

## TOP TIPS FOR GETTING STARTED

Getting started is hard. I understand that. I feel like that every time I have to reset. I feel like I have failed, that I will never get back to my original fitness and that my trainer is judging me. But I promise you that all of that is only in your head. Here are some of my top tips for getting started.

- **Find something you enjoy.** This is vital. Life is too short to be doing an activity you're allergic to. Personally, I'm not a runner (yet – never say never!), so doing that is punishment and I hate it, but I adore the gym and resistance training so it's easier for me to turn up to do that every single day. When you enjoy it, your confidence will rise too.
- **Exercising at your own pace.** Exercise should not hurt you. It should push you and help you grow, not make you vomit.
- **Get checked out by a professional.** If you're worried about your mobility, then make sure you take personal responsibility for it and get advice on what to do safely.
- **Start small and build momentum.** For example, to lose 80 pounds, I went to the gym three times a week for 30 minutes, drank lots of water, increased my NEAT (see page 62) and watched my food.

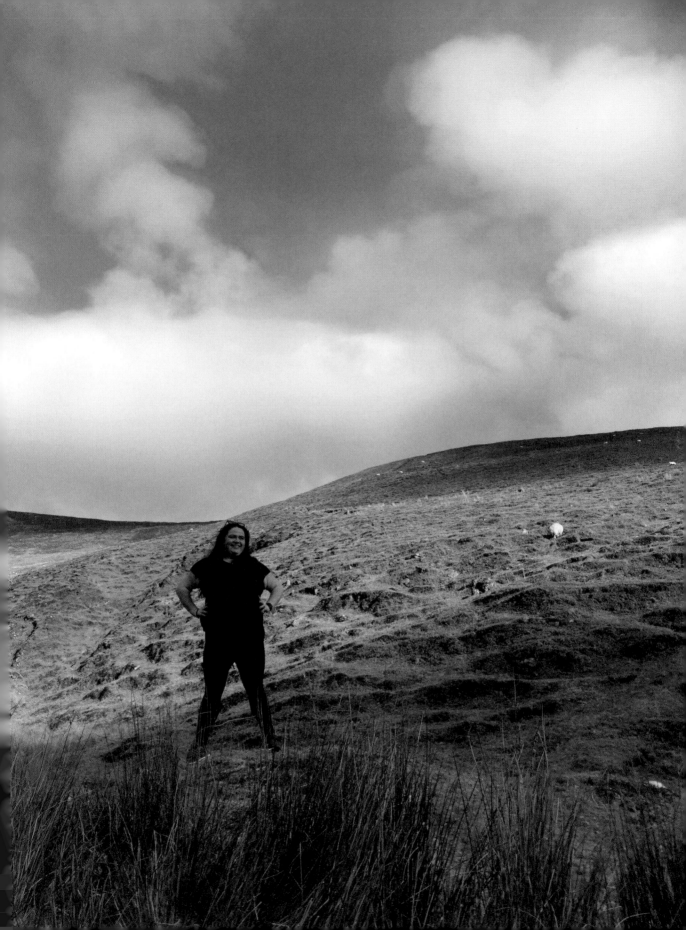

- **Make exercise a routine and a habit.** Try to exercise at the same time on the same days so that time becomes precious to you. I hate working out in the evenings, so instead I make sure it's one of the first things I get done each day.
- **Praise yourself.** Take videos of yourself so that you can see your progress. Make sure you know that you are the one who holds all the power – you can either win at your life or feel bad about not exercising.
- **Choose your suffering.** You can either spend 30 minutes sweating and being pushed out of your comfort zone and the other 23½ hours feeling good or you can spend 24 hours thinking about doing it and putting it off or not bothering at all and feeling guilty.
- **Make it a game.** You vs. you, no one else. Challenge yourself and win every time.
- **Inspire and be inspired.** Fill your ears with podcasts that support your end goal and help you to gain information, then watch as people become inspired by you. You can and you will do this!
- **Cut down on telly.** I know we all love to watch our shows, but try swapping one hour of Netflix or the telly with one hour of exercise instead. That is 365 hours in the year or 15 whole days that you have given your body what it needs: movement.
- **Give yourself rewards.** For every 5 pounds that you lose, buy yourself something that will make your exercise more fun: a smartwatch, headphones, new tops, bottoms, socks and runners. Don't reward yourself with food!

*At first, they may laugh.*
*Then they will ask you how you did it.*

# PODCASTS

The power of a good podcast is amazing. I love them because I can choose what I want to hear. When we turn on the radio or the news these days it can be scary and negative, whereas with a podcast in my ears, I can be in charge of what I listen to. They can be great for listening to for motivation in the gym instead of music. There is nothing better than going for a walk and getting lost in a podcast.

Here's a list of my 10 favourite podcasts that I listen to for laughs or pure escapism or to gain more knowledge for my journey. I've even popped up on a few of these.

1. **The Laughs of Your Life:** One of my favourites for laughing and getting to see other sides of guests. Doireann Garrihy is hilarious herself. I have listened to every single episode and laughed without fail each time. A really great podcast.

2. **Where Is My Mind?:** I adore this podcast for so many reasons. Niall 'Bressie' Breslin addresses some serious topics surrounding mental health and the impact that society has on us all and includes real-life stories from incredible people. It's amazing for mindfulness and meditation. A gem of a pod!

3. **The Brian Keane Podcast:** If you want to really get to know nutrition, exercise and all things health, then this is the podcast for you. Brian is also one of life's gentlemen who does his best to give back and is honest about the fitness world.

4. **The Paul Dermody Podcast:** Paul's message is so clear and his podcast really helps you to understand the health, fitness and weight loss world with amazing analogies. His results speak for themselves.

5. **The 2 Johnnies Podcast:** I have spent so many days roaming around the roads roaring laughing at this podcast. I've never finished an episode not feeling good and uplifted. No matter who they have on to interview, I'm hooked.

6. **An Oral History of the Office:** If, like me, you're a fan of the US version of *The Office*, this little gem will keep you moving.

7. **The Good Glow:** Georgie Crawford is an inspirational woman who has battled breast cancer and has such a wonderful manner when interviewing guests. She brings the best out of her guests and really lets the story be told.

8. **The Joe Rogan Experience:** I usually don't have a clue who the person is who he interviews, but I still find myself hooked on a 3-hour episode.

9. **The Blindboy Podcast:** A diverse, broad mixture of interviews, psychology and comedy. Don't miss the episode with Graham Norton!

10. **The Tommy and Hector Podcast with Laura Blewitt:** My god, I roar laughing listening to this! This is just one that will keep you walking and laughing, which is amazing!

So get your headphones on and get out. Podcasts and exercise are a wonderful combination. Remember, you have control of what you consume and when you consume it.

## SCALES AND MEASURING YOUR PROGRESS

I've called the scale many names when the number it gave me didn't match what I felt. It was wrong, it was a bully, blah blah blah. What I have since learned is that I was attaching too much emotion to the scale. The scale is purely data. If you are morbidly obese like me, that data is a helpful indicator of how you're getting on, but I've learned from Brian Keane and Paul Dermody that the scale is a tool for measuring weight loss, but it doesn't show you fat loss.

Weight loss and fat loss are two different things. Losing body fat means your shape is changing and you are chipping away at fat. This will happen when you have the 25:25:25:25 rules down to a T! Losing weight is the number on the scale. Losing both fat and weight is the magic moment you know that you are on track and your body composition is changing.

When the scale doesn't move you may be losing body fat while gaining muscle, so don't fire the baby out with the bathwater. You need to remove the emotion of looking at the scale, not agreeing with the figure and reacting like a child by hitting the self-sabotage button. If you come off the scale and aren't happy with the number, just move on with your day and stay in the reset mode. Consistency will win. The scale will have no option but to move in time.

But I understand how it can ruin your day, if not your week. It's normal to feel disheartened when your weight is up and happier when your weight is down. Just focus on adapting and changing into a healthier lifestyle. If you are on and off the scale numerous times a day, your relationship with it may be toxic. In that case, you have to take control, set a boundary and manage it. Ask yourself, 'If I hop on the scale, am I going to be okay with the result even if it's up?' As a responsible adult, you should know if you're in the right frame of mind or not. The solution may even be to dump it, which is what I had to do. Now I weigh in every few weeks on the machine in the local chemist.

Instead of relying solely on the scale, I also use pictures, measurements and my own feelings (if I feel good, I'm doing good!) to know when I'm progressing. I know how much you hate photos. I know how scared you are of being tagged in photos from a night out. But trust me when I say this: take the photo now. Get into that bra and knickers and get the photo done, because someday that hero in that photo will be your before picture, and you owe it to that person to have documented who they were.

And remember, the scale doesn't account for everything. Focus on your happiness, your energy levels and the things you love. The weight will come off you if you follow this approach. Weight loss is simply a positive side effect of true health, happiness, self-love and inner peace

## WEIGHT LOSS AND PERIODS

If you are like me and you have lost your periods then take this as a sign to go and get it checked with a doctor. I lost mine for years when I was really gaining the weight. Thankfully they have come back. If you listen to my episode on the *Laughs of Your Life* podcast with Doireann Garrihy, you will hear the story of when and where they came back. Also now I have noticed that on the week it is due and when I am on it, it is so much harder to get the scales to move and I am more tired and bloated, but we're all different. My advice here is to listen to your own body and to take a rest if you need to.

## NEAT: NATURALLY EXERCISE AND TRANSFORM

What is NEAT and why do people always bring it up? It's a real term – non-exercise activity thermogenesis – but I like to call it naturally exercise and transform. I think of it as sneaking in extra movement all day without getting out of breath or sweaty. In my mind, this is the activity and calories burned outside of my workout: my walking, housework, shopping, hoovering. Whenever your body moves it's burning calories, and the more you burn, the more weight you lose.

Here are my top NEAT tips on becoming more aware of your body and making it move more. All these add to your NEAT and inevitably help you to hit your goals that little bit more easily.

- **Invest in a standing desk,** as even just standing still burns calories.
- **Play with your kids** for 20 minutes a day.
- **Go for a 30-minute walk outside** – 15 minutes one way and 15 minutes back.
- **Take the stairs** instead of the lift.
- **Invest in a smartwatch** and set yourself challenges.
- **Park further away from the front door of the supermarket.** (If you're like me, you nearly drive into the store!)
- **If possible, walk to the shop** instead of driving.
- **Do some housework** and make sure you are moving well.
- **Dance around the kitchen** while the spuds are boiling!

These are all very simple habits that you can add to your day and they won't change it majorly, but they will benefit you in the long run. I promise you that after moving more each day over the course of a year, you will be a different person. As the saying goes, 'Tell me what you do every day and I will tell you where you are in a year.'

Keep figuring out ways that will enrich your body and your mind. Remember, the more you move, the better your mood. You can do this. You can move more. You may not want to, but you know you should. Give your body what it needs and desires: movement and feeling good.

# 25: Nutrition

## NUTRITIONAL INFORMATION

For this book I decided to include calories and macros. I'm still not doing a regime of strict counting, as having BED means that I can struggle with strictness, so instead I eat intuitively and focus on learning when I'm full. But the calories and macros are a helpful tool and I do like to know how many calories are in the food that I'm eating, plus I know that a lot of people count calories and I wanted to make sure that my second book suits everyone. Sometimes you can think that you're eating something healthy but it could be very high in fat or calories, so this is just another tool for you to use to manage your lifestyle better. Knowledge is power and it's a good idea to be aware of the number of calories in food.

## HOW TO PLAN YOUR MEALS

I always plan my meals just before I go to the supermarket. I'm a brand ambassador for Aldi, so I do all my shopping there and I just love it for quality and price. I plan my meals with a biro and a piece of paper. I sit down on the day that I do my weekly shop (usually a Sunday) and write down what I will have Monday through to Sunday. I often plan my meals using a list or a grid – see page 72 for my 21-Day Reset sample meal plan.

Once I've planned my meals for the week, I write down what I will need to create seven days' worth of those dishes and only buy that. Once you have a list, it's much easier and faster to do your shop. Making a list also means you spend less money and have less empty calories! So on page 64 is what my shopping list would be for the week of meals (although a lot of these are store cupboard staples that I wouldn't need to buy every week).

# TRISHA'S SHOPPING LIST

**FRESH FRUIT, VEG AND HERBS:**
- [ ] Bananas
- [ ] Lemons
- [ ] Limes
- [ ] Button mushrooms
- [ ] Carrots
- [ ] Celery
- [ ] Flat mushrooms
- [ ] Garlic
- [ ] Ginger or ginger purée
- [ ] Green beans
- [ ] Green and red chillies
- [ ] Mangetout
- [ ] Maris Piper potatoes
- [ ] Onions (white and red)
- [ ] Shallots
- [ ] Spring onions
- [ ] Basil
- [ ] Chives
- [ ] Coriander
- [ ] Flat-leaf parsley
- [ ] Lemongrass
- [ ] Rosemary
- [ ] Thyme

**MEAT:**
- [ ] Boneless, skinless chicken breasts
- [ ] Prime cut of beef, such as sirloin or fillet
- [ ] Streaky bacon

**CUPBOARD:**
- [ ] Olive oil
- [ ] Sesame oil
- [ ] Basmati rice
- [ ] Caster sugar
- [ ] Chicken and vegetable stock cubes
- [ ] Honey
- [ ] Lighter-than-light mayonnaise
- [ ] Oats
- [ ] Plain flour
- [ ] Reduced-fat coconut milk
- [ ] Tinned tuna
- [ ] Tins of chopped tomatoes
- [ ] Tomato purée

**FRIDGE AND FREEZER:**
- [ ] Eggs
- [ ] Breadcrumbs
- [ ] Butter
- [ ] Low-fat milk
- [ ] Low-fat natural yoghurt
- [ ] 0% fat Greek yoghurt
- [ ] Light cream
- [ ] Reduced-fat crème fraîche
- [ ] Light red Cheddar cheese
- [ ] Feta cheese
- [ ] Frozen petit pois

**SPICES:**
- [ ] Cayenne pepper
- [ ] Garam masala
- [ ] Garlic powder
- [ ] Ground cinnamon
- [ ] Ground coriander
- [ ] Ground cumin
- [ ] Lime leaves
- [ ] Paprika (smoked and regular)
- [ ] Shrimp paste
- [ ] Salt and black pepper

# DOING THE 'BIG SHOP'

- **Make your menu, then make your shopping list.** Yes, I'm repeating myself, but this is important. You will waste time and money without these. When you run out of something, pop it into the notes on your phone so that you remember to get it in the next shop.

- **Organise your list by the aisles.** I know from looking at my list the exact route that I take around the shop.

- **Do a stock check.** Check your fridge and presses before you leave and cross the stuff off the list that you already have to prevent overbuying.

- **Don't go shopping hungry.** You will only make poor decisions and buy stuff you don't want or need.

- **Remember NEAT.** Park as far away from the door as possible to add to your NEAT. Or even better, leave the car at home and walk to the shop if you can.

- **Buy frozen to get ahead.** Buy frozen chopped onions, garlic, chilli and ginger to save time on prep.

- **Look for specials.** See if you can adapt your list to include items that are on special offer. For example, if you need chicken breasts and chicken strips are on offer, go with them. However, if a special offer is on and you don't need it and it's not on your list, do not buy it!

- **Only buy food in your supermarket.** Remember my diesel diet? Make it a rule to never buy food in garages.

- **Check the dates.** If you're batch cooking, make sure the use by or best before dates all have a five-day lead time.

- **Go for leaner cuts of meat.** Ask your butcher to take the skin or the fat off in advance so that it removes the temptation of having it at home.

- **Buy seasonal.** Food is more nutritious and tastes better when you buy it in season. Plus you'll get it when it's at its peak production, which is also when it's cheapest.

- **Buy cooked meats.** If you think that you may not have time, then purchase cooked chicken, etc.

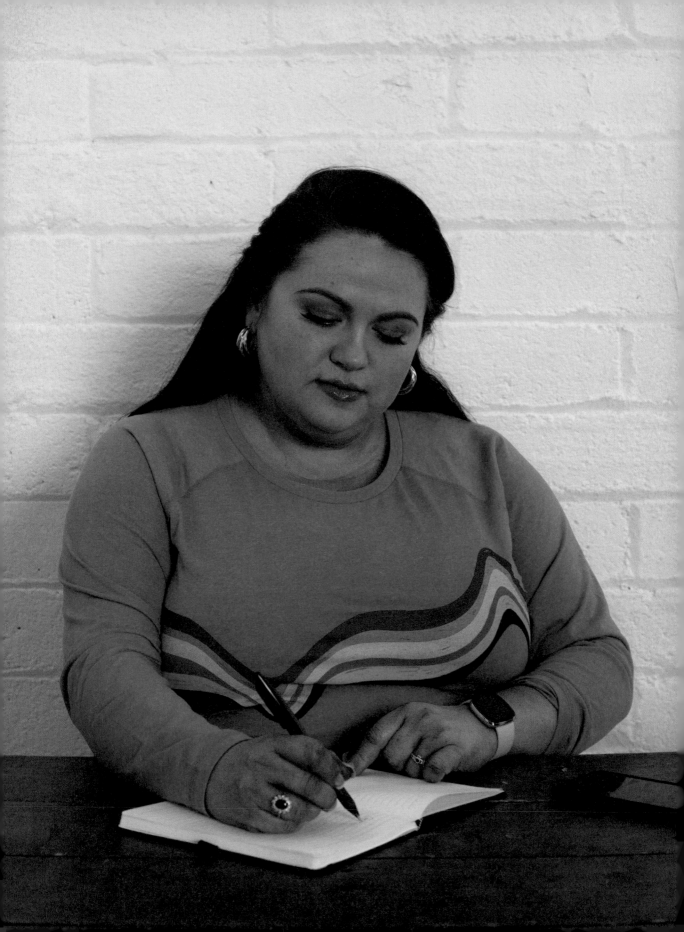

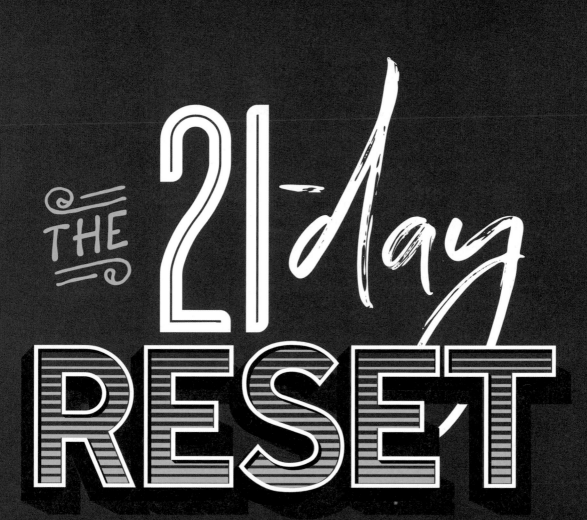

# THE 21-day RESET

YOU HAVE 21 DAYS - JUST THREE WEEKS.
ARE YOU READY TO KICK OFF
THE BEST TIME OF YOUR LIFE?

# WHY THREE WEEKS?

Three weeks is your short-term goal. So every three weeks, you start again – do this 17 times and you'll have completed a year of resets for a happier, healthier you! After every three-week cycle, look back on your previous work and see what you can improve on. Chart your progress using the table on page 77.

The reason I do my resets in three-week cycles is because it's so manageable. If you find that you're struggling, you know that a reset is on the way, so keep going. Always remember it is day by day and pound by pound. You can only manage the manageables!

Start seeing resetting not as a bad thing but as a tool to get you to your end goal and to see what you can remove or improve on.

On page 10, you wrote down your long-term goal. So, for example, if that goal was to lose four stone, your short-term 21-day goal would be to lose 3 lbs in three weeks. If you do this consistently for 17 resets, you will have gotten rid of 51 lbs. The goal of losing four stone becomes a lot less scary when you break it down.

**Make a goal for this reset and fill it in here:**

.........................................................................................................................................................

Think about what you want to achieve, how you are going to achieve it and the curveballs you see coming.

# IT IS NEVER TOO LATE TO BE WHO YOU SHOULD HAVE BEEN

# MY WEEKLY RESET PLANS

**Thought/quote of the week**

I love motivational quotes as they provide with me with a quick burst of wisdom that helps me get my focus back. When you are lacking motivation, a quote can inspire you and help you get back on track.

**My goal for this week**

When you are setting goals, always set SMART goals. SMART goals are specific, measurable, attainable, relevant and time-bound.

- **Specific.** Don't beat around the bush here – what is your goal for this week? If you want to lose 3 lbs over the course of this 21-day reset, your goal for this week could be to lose just 1 lb.
- **Measureable.** How will I track it? It can be the scales, pictures, inches or energy.
- **Attainable.** You need to look at your history here. Why have I stopped in the past? How can I prevent this? Always remember that once a goal has been hit you can set a new one straight away and just keep pushing for the end goal – happiness!
- **Relevant.** It needs to matter to your life for you to achieve it. I know that if I stay the same weight or gain more that is relevant enough to affect my life. Keep reminding yourself of the reasons you are doing this when you want to quit!
- **Time-bound.** Never adjust the specific goal but you may need to adjust the time. That is why the 21-day reset is so handy, as every three weeks is an end date and a start date!

## 25: NUTRITION

At the start of each week, I want you to create a meal plan for the next seven days. Batch cooking will be key here, as will a good shopping list so that you buy only what you need. My personal preference is to have the same thing for a couple of days in a row, as it keeps me on track. I generally have the same thing Monday to Friday, then I change it up for the weekend. But you do not have to copy me. Always remember that this is your lifestyle, so it has to suit you! Your goal for the week should be – and must be – a non-negotiable.

## 25: WATER

During the day, track how much water you drink by crossing off a droplet. Each droplet represents 250ml.

## 25: EXERCISE

At the start of each week, plan your exercise. Take into account that not every day can be 15k steps.

## 25: SLEEP

Every morning, record when you went to sleep and when you got up. You would always recharge your phone so you have to look at that for yourself too. Smartwatches are amazing but I find you can become nearly obsessive about checking how much you slept. If you want data, write down what time you went to sleep and when you woke. Having a routine is key here, so try and aim for the same bedtime each night for consistency!

## WHAT I DON'T WANT TO REPEAT

At the end of the week, take a look at what didn't go so well. Did you not drink enough water? Did you give out about yourself in a mean way? Did the scales not move and you hit the self-sabotage button? Did you eat food secretly and dump the wrappers? Did you have guilt that you shouldn't have with food? Was your screen-time too high?

## WHAT I WANT TO TAKE FORWARD

At the end of the week, give yourself credit for the amazing work you've done this week. What made you smile? What made you proud? What did you prove to yourself that you could do after all this time telling yourself you couldn't? What was fun? How much better do you feel in comparison to last week?

# TRISHA'S WEEKLY PLAN

| THOUGHT/QUOTE OF THE WEEK | If your dreams do not scare you, they are not big enough. |
|---|---|
| MY GOAL FOR THIS WEEK | Go to the gym three times and get at least 7 hours of sleep every night. |

**25: Nutrition**

| | | Monday | Tuesday | Wednesday | Thursday | Friday | Saturday | Sunday |
|---|---|---|---|---|---|---|---|---|
| Nutrition | Breakfast | Cinnamon and banana porridge Page 80 | Cinnamon and banana porridge Page 80 | Cinnamon and banana porridge Page 80 | Cinnamon and banana porridge Page 80 | Cinnamon and banana porridge Page 80 | Cinnamon and banana porridge Page 80 | Shakshuka Page 88 |
| | Lunch | Mushroom soup Page 108 | Mushroom soup Page 108 | Mushroom soup Page 108 | Mushroom soup Page 108 | Mushroom soup Page 108 | Tuna melts Page 121 | Roast beef (I have my dinner early on Sunday) Page 128 |
| | Dinner | Thai green chicken curry Page 136 | Thai green chicken curry Page 136 | Thai green chicken curry Page 136 | Thai green chicken curry Page 136 | Thai green chicken curry Page 136 | Indian butter chicken Page 138 | Spicy potato wedges with whipped feta Page 181, 174 |
| 25: | Water | 💧💧💧💧💧💧💧💧 | 💧💧💧💧💧💧💧 | 💧💧💧💧💧💧 | 💧💧💧💧💧💧💧 | 💧💧💧💧💧💧💧💧 | 💧💧💧💧💧💧💧💧 | 💧💧💧💧💧💧💧 |
| 25: | Exercise | MOVE: 30-minute walk (breathless) | REST DAY: 20-minute stroll | NEAT: 30-minute walk | GYM: Legs | GYM: Back and shoulders | REST DAY: 20-minute stroll | NEAT: 30-minute walk or a class |
| 25: | Sleep | 10 p.m. to 6 a.m | 10 p.m. to 7 a.m. | 11 p.m. to 7 a.m. | 10:30 p.m. to 9 a.m. | 11 p.m. to 8 a.m. | 11 p.m. to 9 a.m. | 11 p.m. to 8 a.m. |

| What I don't want to repeat | I missed the gym on Thursday and was very hard on myself about it. But I know that next week is a brand new week and I can start again! I have learned from this week that I still struggle to say no and when an excuse arises I jump at the opportunity. |
|---|---|
| What I want to take forward | I can feel a big difference in my energy levels. I feel tired but I can also say that I feel content that I pushed myself to be a better version of me. |

# YOUR 21-DAY RESET: WEEK ONE

| | THOUGHT/QUOTE OF THE WEEK | | | | | | |
|---|---|---|---|---|---|---|---|
| | MY GOAL FOR THIS WEEK | | | | | | |

| | | Monday | Tuesday | Wednesday | Thursday | Friday | Saturday | Sunday |
|---|---|---|---|---|---|---|---|---|
| **25: Nutrition** | Breakfast | | | | | | | |
| | Lunch | | | | | | | |
| | Dinner | | | | | | | |
| **25:** | Water | ◊◊◊◊◊◊◊◊ | ◊◊◊◊◊◊◊◊ | ◊◊◊◊◊◊◊◊ | ◊◊◊◊◊◊◊◊ | ◊◊◊◊◊◊◊◊ | ◊◊◊◊◊◊◊◊ | ◊◊◊◊◊◊◊◊ |
| **25:** | Exercise | | | | | | | |
| **25:** | Sleep | | | | | | | |
| | What I don't want to repeat | | | | | | | |
| | What I want to take forward | | | | | | | |

# WEEK TWO

| THOUGHT/QUOTE OF THE WEEK | | | | | | | |
|---|---|---|---|---|---|---|---|
| **MY GOAL FOR THIS WEEK** | | | | | | | |
| | Monday | Tuesday | Wednesday | Thursday | Friday | Saturday | Sunday |
| Breakfast | | | | | | | |
| Lunch | | | | | | | |
| Dinner | | | | | | | |
| Water | | | | | | | |
| Exercise | | | | | | | |
| Sleep | | | | | | | |
| What I don't want to repeat | | | | | | | |
| What I want to take forward | | | | | | | |

25: **Nutrition**

25:

25:

25:

# WEEK THREE

| | **THOUGHT/QUOTE OF THE WEEK** | | | | | | |
|---|---|---|---|---|---|---|---|
| | **MY GOAL FOR THIS WEEK** | | | | | | |

| | Monday | Tuesday | Wednesday | Thursday | Friday | Saturday | Sunday |
|---|---|---|---|---|---|---|---|
| **Breakfast** | | | | | | | |
| **Lunch** | | | | | | | |
| **Dinner** | | | | | | | |
| **Water** | 🌢🌢🌢🌢🌢🌢🌢🌢 | 🌢🌢🌢🌢🌢🌢🌢🌢 | 🌢🌢🌢🌢🌢🌢🌢🌢 | 🌢🌢🌢🌢🌢🌢🌢🌢 | 🌢🌢🌢🌢🌢🌢🌢🌢 | 🌢🌢🌢🌢🌢🌢🌢🌢 | 🌢🌢🌢🌢🌢🌢🌢🌢 |
| **Exercise** | | | | | | | |
| **Sleep** | | | | | | | |

**25: Nutrition**

**25:**

**25:**

**25:**

| | | | | | | | |
|---|---|---|---|---|---|---|---|
| **What I don't want to repeat** | | | | | | | |
| **What I want to take forward** | | | | | | | |

## THE RESET REFLECTION

**At the end of every three-week reset, reflect on these questions.**

- How are you feeling?

- Was it easier than you thought?

- Was it harder than you thought?

- Do you feel lighter mentally?

- Did you do your weekly shop?

- What dish did you learn how to make?

- Did you enjoy batch cooking?

- Did you increase your movement?

- Did you drink more water?

- What can you improve on for the next three weeks?

- What is your goal for three weeks from now?

- What was not sustainable?

- What can you replace that with instead?

- Do you feel good?

- Are you proud of yourself?

- What was your favourite part?

- What have you learned about yourself?

- What are you excited for in the next reset?

- Are you ready to go again?

## PROGRESS CHART

Tick off the weeks as you complete each of your reset cycles and remember to keep track of your achievements for each reset. Remember, 17 of these three-week cycles equals one year.

| | Week 1 | Week 2 | Week 3 | Achievement |
|---|---|---|---|---|
| Reset 1 | | | | |
| Reset 2 | | | | |
| Reset 3 | | | | |
| Reset 4 | | | | |
| Reset 5 | | | | |
| Reset 6 | | | | |
| Reset 7 | | | | |
| Reset 8 | | | | |
| Reset 9 | | | | |
| Reset 10 | | | | |
| Reset 11 | | | | |
| Reset 12 | | | | |
| Reset 13 | | | | |
| Reset 14 | | | | |
| Reset 15 | | | | |
| Reset 16 | | | | |
| Reset 17 | | | | |

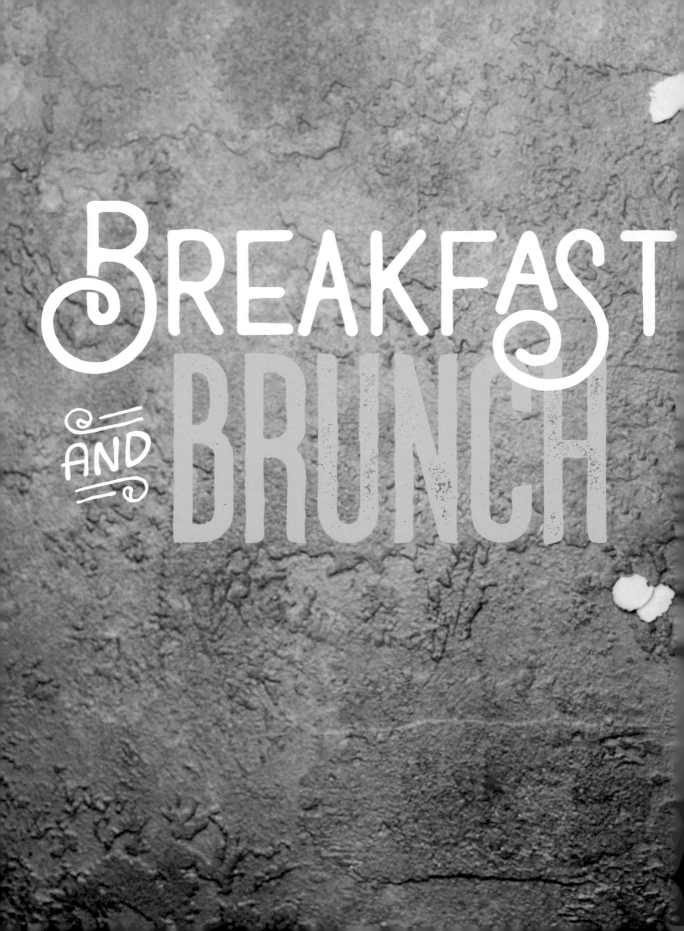

# Breakfast

## AND

# BRUNCH

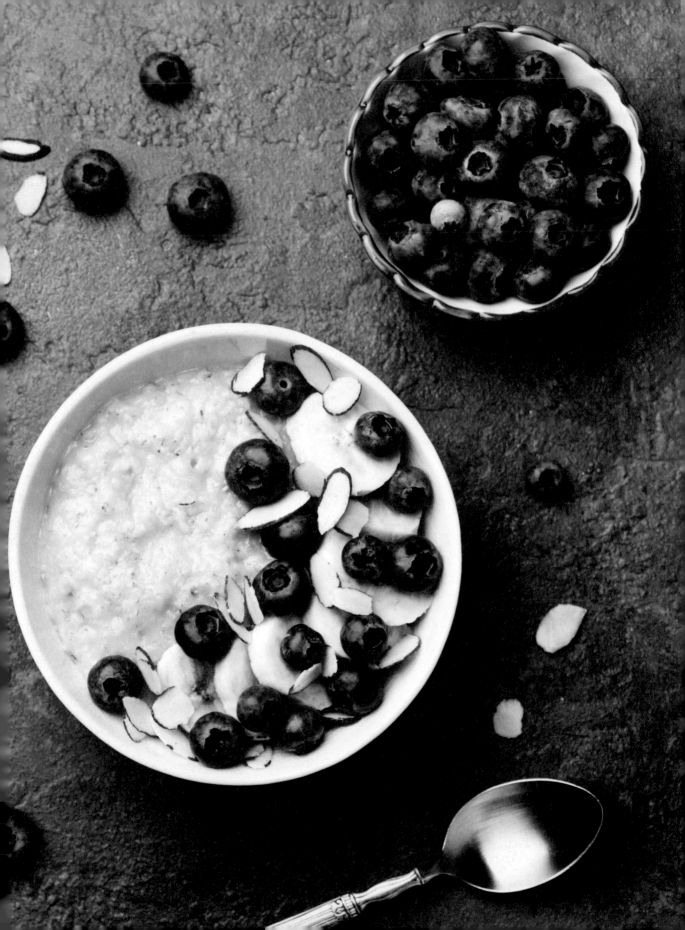

# CINNAMON AND BANANA PORRIDGE

Porridge is a comfort food; it's like a warm hug first thing in the morning.
It also gives you the fuel that you will need for a busy day. It's cheap, nutritious and filling
and the best thing is that oats are a very neutral flavour, so you can have so much fun
with the flavour combinations.

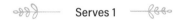 Serves 1

170ml low-fat milk

35g oats

20g low-fat natural yoghurt

1 medium banana, sliced

1 tsp ground cinnamon

drizzle of honey

Pour your milk into a pot and bring to the boil. Add your oats, reduce the heat and stir continuously. After 4 minutes, your oats should be ready. Stir in your natural yoghurt and pour the porridge into a bowl.

To serve, scatter over your banana, sprinkle your cinnamon on top and drizzle over your honey.

**Nutritional Information**

|  | Per Serving |
| --- | --- |
| Calories | 359kcal |
| Protein | 12g |
| Carbohydrates | 62g |
| Fat | 7g |
| Vegetarian | ✔ |

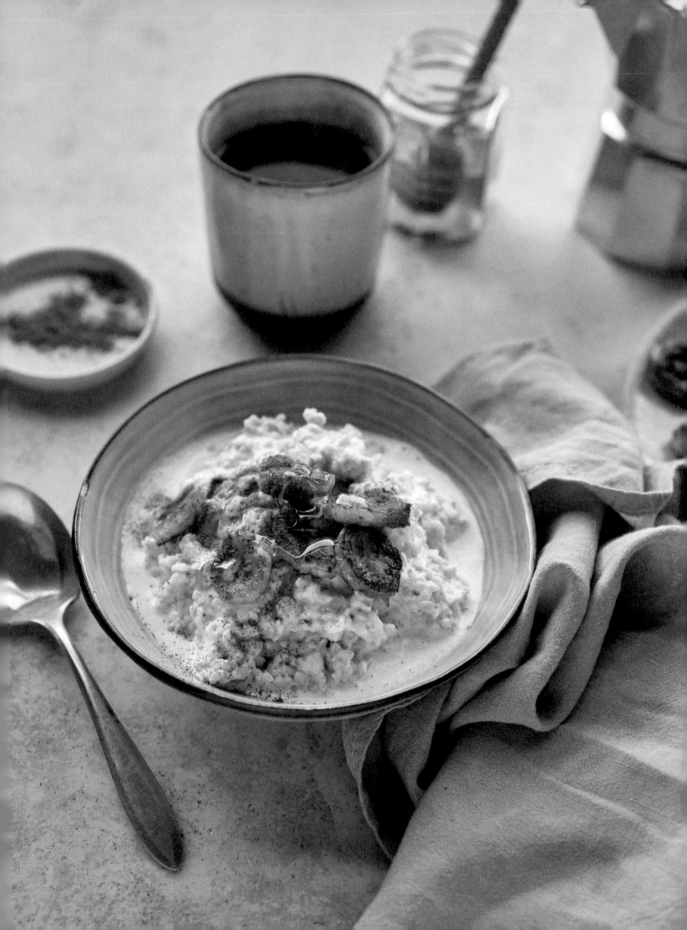

# OVERNIGHT BERRY AND NUT BUTTER OATS

This is so handy if you are short on time in the morning,
as you can make this two days in advance. This breakfast will give
you slow-releasing energy for the day.

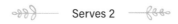 Serves 2

100g oats

200ml low-fat milk

¼ tsp ground cinnamon

pinch of salt

60g low-fat natural yoghurt

100g fresh berries

1 tbsp peanut butter (or any
nut butter, but avoid ones
with palm oil)

drizzle of honey

Stir together your oats, milk, cinnamon and salt. Pour
into two glasses and pop in the fridge overnight.

The next day, stir the oats and add some extra milk if
needed. To serve, spoon your yoghurt, berries and nut
butter on top and drizzle with honey.

**Nutritional Information**

|  | Per Serving |
| --- | --- |
| Calories | 340kcal |
| Protein | 14g |
| Carbohydrates | 46g |
| Fat | 10g |
| Vegetarian | ✔ |

# APPLE AND CINNAMON OAT PANCAKES

These pancakes are packed with nutrients, but still feel like a treat. These are easy to make, as you can make the batter ahead of time and have it ready in the fridge. You can change the combinations, but I'm old school and apple and cinnamon just rocks! These are also a lovely option to have after a workout, as these pancakes are full of protein and complex carbohydrates to allow your body to refuel and recover.

Serves 1

With a NutriBullet or high-speed blender, blitz your oats and cinnamon into a fine powder. Pour into a bowl with your apple, beaten eggs, oat milk and sweetener and stir to combine into a batter.

Heat a non-stick frying pan and add some low-calorie cooking spray. Make sure the pan is clean and not too hot, otherwise the pancakes will stick or burn. Spoon 2 tablespoons of batter into the pan and let it cook for at least 1 minute, then flip over and finish cooking on the other side.

Serve with some yoghurt and an extra sprinkle of cinnamon. Strawberries work well as a garnish when they're in season.

60g oats
½ tsp ground cinnamon, plus extra to serve
1 apple, peeled, cored and diced into tiny cubes
3 eggs, beaten
75ml oat milk
1½ tsp Canderel sweetener
low-calorie cooking spray
low-fat natural yoghurt, to serve

**Nutritional Information**

|  | Per Serving |
| --- | --- |
| Calories | 291kcal |
| Protein | 16g |
| Carbohydrates | 24g |
| Fat | 14g |
| Vegetarian | ✔ |

# RASPBERRY AND VANILLA BAKED OATS

Baked oats are so handy. They are filling and packed with fibre, which is ideal when you're trying to get the scales to tip in the right direction! Serving these straight from the oven with a mug of tea is such a nutritious but fun way to start the day. Often if I'm going on a long walk or hike, I will leave this to cool then chop it up into squares so that I can have some snacks on the way.

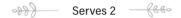 Serves 2

low-calorie cooking spray

200g low-fat natural yoghurt, plus extra to serve

60g raspberries, plus extra to serve

50g oats

2 large or 3 medium eggs

1½ tsp vanilla extract

Preheat your oven to 200°C. Grease a small baking tin or ovenproof dish with some low-calorie cooking spray.

This is a one-bowl wonder. Literally put everything into the bowl and mix together, then pour into your greased tin and bake in the preheated oven for 35 minutes.

To serve, add a spoonful of yoghurt on top, then scatter over a few fresh raspberries for a pop of colour.

**Nutritional Information**

| | Per Serving |
|---|---|
| Calories | 279kcal |
| Protein | 16g |
| Carbohydrates | 28g |
| Fat | 11g |
| Vegetarian | ✔ |

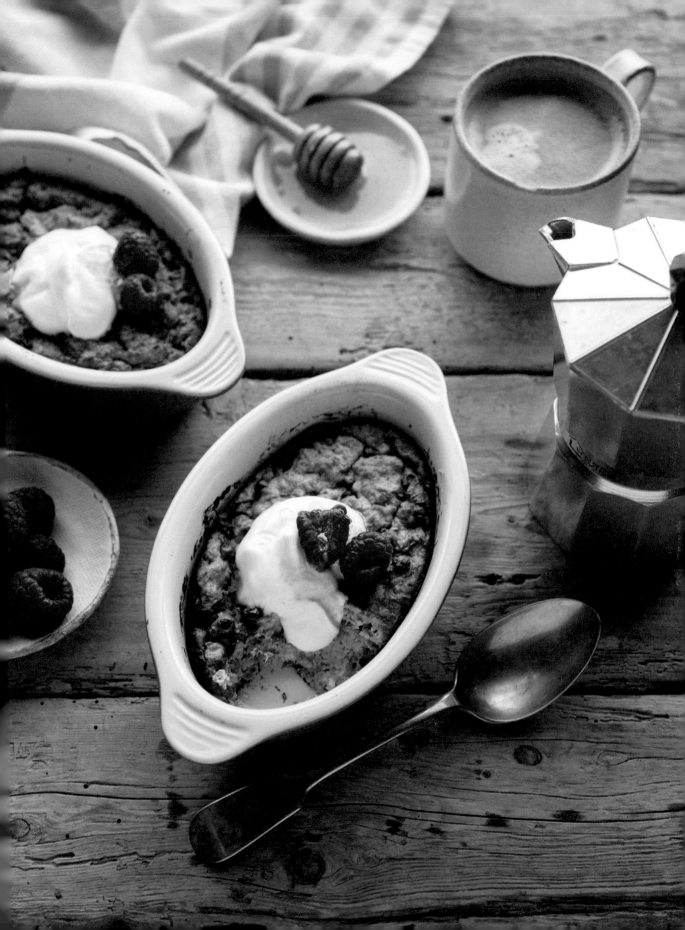

# HOMEMADE HASH BROWNS
## WITH STREAKY BACON AND POACHED EGGS

This dish requires very few ingredients and very little effort to make – easy but impressive! Hash browns are very similar to potato rösti. Pop a poached egg on top and away you go. A few slices of avocado on the side are a nice extra but would increase the fat. Hash browns can be quite bland, so make sure you season them well. The saltiness of the bacon will also enhance the flavour.

Serves 4

6 medium potatoes (Maris Pipers work best here)
salt and black pepper
2 small white onions, finely diced
2 eggs, beaten
olive oil, for cooking
100g streaky bacon
poached eggs, to serve
fresh chives, to garnish

Using the coarse side of a box grater, grate your potatoes onto a baking tray. Sprinkle 1 teaspoon of salt over the grated potatoes, then push them all to one edge of the tray. Pop your tray on a slant so that the potatoes are on the top and all the water is dripping to the bottom.

Let them sit like this for 20 minutes, then place your potatoes into a clean tea towel and squeeze out all the extra water. The key here is to make sure that your potato mixture is really dry so that the hash browns hold their shape when you cook them.

Preheat your grill.

Put the grated potatoes in a bowl with your diced onions and beaten eggs and season well with salt and pepper, as hash browns can be quite bland otherwise. Divide the mixture into four portions.

Heat a non-stick pan and add your olive oil. Add the hash brown portions, working in batches if needed, and fry until golden brown on each side.

Meanwhile, grill your bacon until crispy and poach your eggs, one per person.

Serve the hash browns with the crispy bacon and a poached egg on top, then garnish with fresh chives.

## Nutritional Information

|  | Per Serving |
| --- | --- |
| Calories | 486kcal |
| Protein | 25g |
| Carbohydrates | 45g |
| Fat | 22g |
| Gluten Free | ✔ |

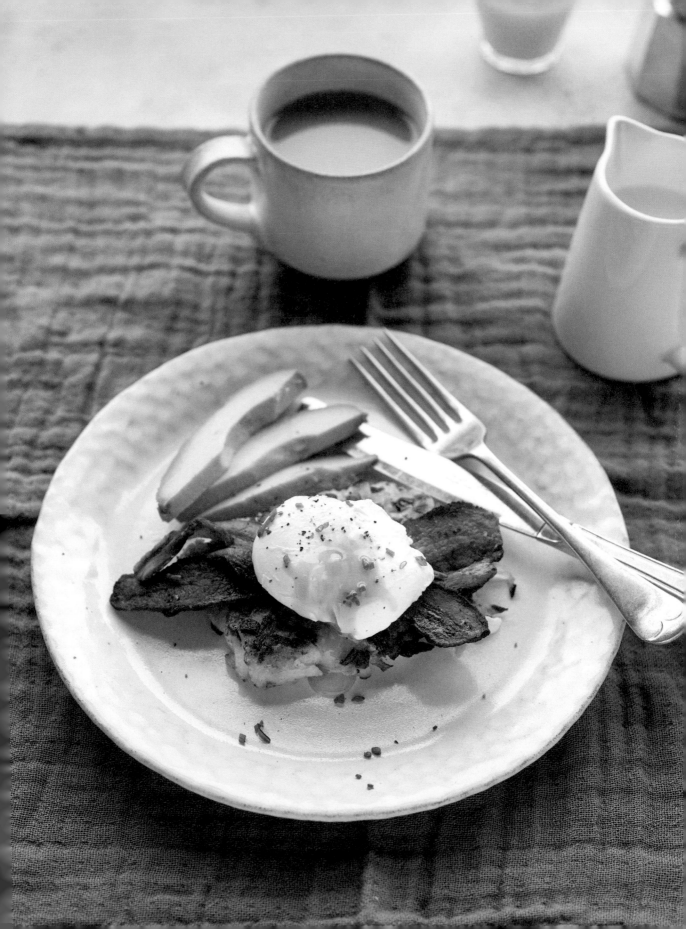

# SHAKSHUKA

This is an ideal one-pot wonder for brunch that looks amazing,
is low in calories and simply delicious. A nice one to suit all the family.

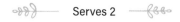 Serves 2

olive oil

2 red onions, diced

1 garlic clove, crushed

1 fresh red chilli, diced

20g fresh coriander, chopped (reserve a few whole leaves to garnish)

2 x 400g tins of chopped tomatoes

50ml water

1 tsp caster sugar

salt and black pepper

4 eggs

crusty bread, to serve

Heat a frying pan and add your olive oil. Add your onions, garlic, chilli and coriander and sauté until the onions are softened.

Add your chopped tomatoes, water and sugar and simmer for 10 minutes. Season well with salt and pepper.

Make four wells in the tomato mixture and crack an egg into each well. Put a lid on your pan and simmer until the eggs are cooked to your liking. I usually go for 6 minutes for a softer egg.

Scatter some whole fresh coriander leaves on top to garnish and serve with crusty bread (or not if you want to keep this gluten free).

## Nutritional Information

|  | Per Serving |
| --- | --- |
| Calories | 390kcal |
| Protein | 22g |
| Carbohydrates | 23g |
| Fat | 23g |
| Vegetarian | ✔ |
| Gluten Free | ✔ |

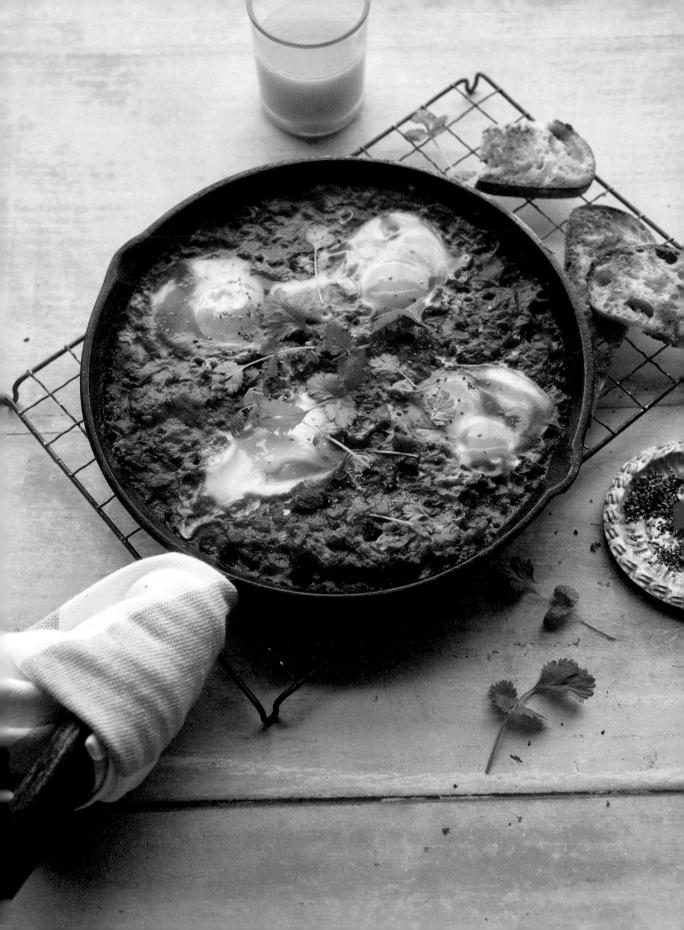

# GREEN EGGS AND HAM

Dr Seuss's most famous dish! I didn't dye the ham, but the eggs are bursting with the green colour from the natural chlorophyll in the kale. This dish is high in protein, which keeps you fuller for longer. Protein is also necessary for growth and repair, which makes this a dish that you could have after exercise. Kale is high in fibre, calcium, vitamins C and K and iron. Serve with a slice of toasted sourdough bread on the side, but this would increase the carbs.

Serves 2

5 cubes of frozen kale, defrosted
2 slices of ham, fat removed
4 eggs
2 egg whites
1 tbsp low-fat milk
salt and black pepper
1 tsp butter
2 spring onions, chopped
2 garlic cloves, finely chopped
fresh flat-leaf parsley leaves, to garnish
½ tsp chilli flakes, to garnish (optional)

Defrost your kale the night before or pop it in the microwave until thawed.

Preheat your grill, then grill your ham until crisp. Set aside.

Meanwhile, whisk together your eggs, egg whites, milk and some salt and pepper in a large bowl, then stir in the thawed kale.

Melt the butter in a frying pan, then add the spring onions and garlic and gently sauté until softened. Add your egg mixture and cook gently until scrambled.

To serve, plate up the eggs with the ham and sprinkle with a few fresh parsley leaves and the chilli flakes (if using).

### Nutritional Information

|  | Per Serving |
| --- | --- |
| Calories | 446kcal |
| Protein | 50g |
| Carbohydrates | 4g |
| Fat | 25g |
| Gluten Free | ✔ |

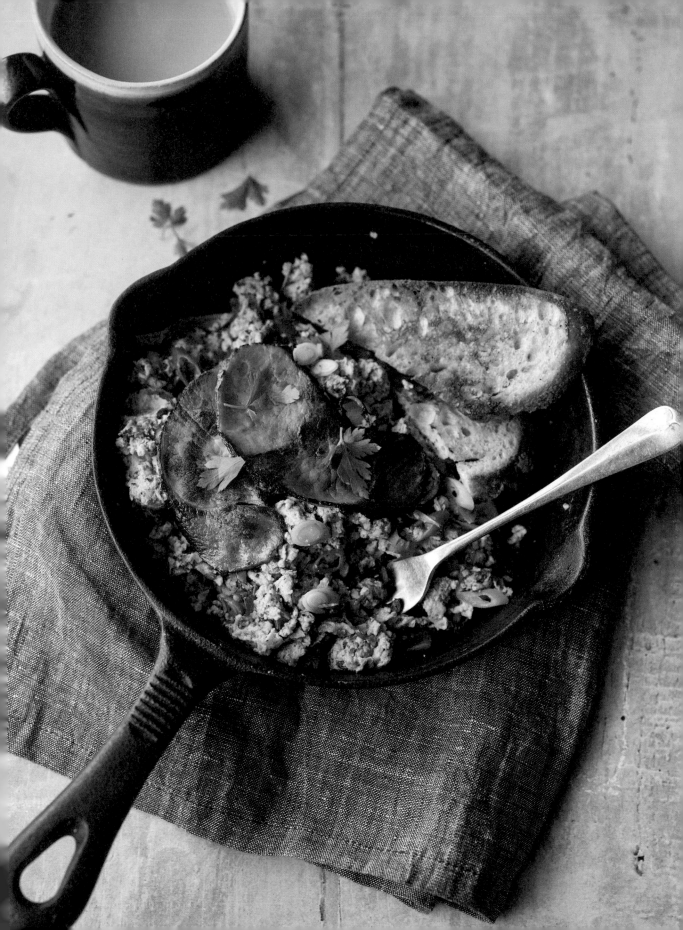

# SPICY SCRAMBLED EGGS
## WITH FETA CHEESE, FENNEL AND CRÈME FRAÎCHE

I first had a version of this in Póg in Dublin and I wanted to make it again and again.
It's so delicious and just bursting with flavour and fun!

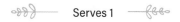 Serves 1

3 medium eggs

2 tsp low-fat milk

1 tsp paprika

1 tsp ground turmeric

1 tsp chilli flakes

15g dry-cured chorizo, chopped

1 spring onion, thinly sliced

1 garlic clove, chopped

25g shredded fennel

15g feta cheese, crumbled

2 tsp reduced-fat crème fraîche

sprig of fresh dill, to garnish

Put your eggs, milk, paprika, turmeric and chilli flakes in a bowl and whisk together.

Heat a frying pan, then add your chopped chorizo. There's no need to add any oil, as the oil in the chorizo will come out as it cooks. Add the spring onion and garlic and gently fry until the chorizo is cooked through. Pour in your egg mixture and gently scramble. I always cook my eggs with a spatula, as it doesn't break them up and keeps them fluffy.

Spoon onto a plate and scatter over the fennel and feta, then spoon the crème fraîche on top and garnish with a little fresh dill.

### Nutritional Information

|  | Per Serving |
| --- | --- |
| Calories | 457kcal |
| Protein | 30g |
| Carbohydrates | 15g |
| Fat | 29g |
| Gluten Free | ✔ |

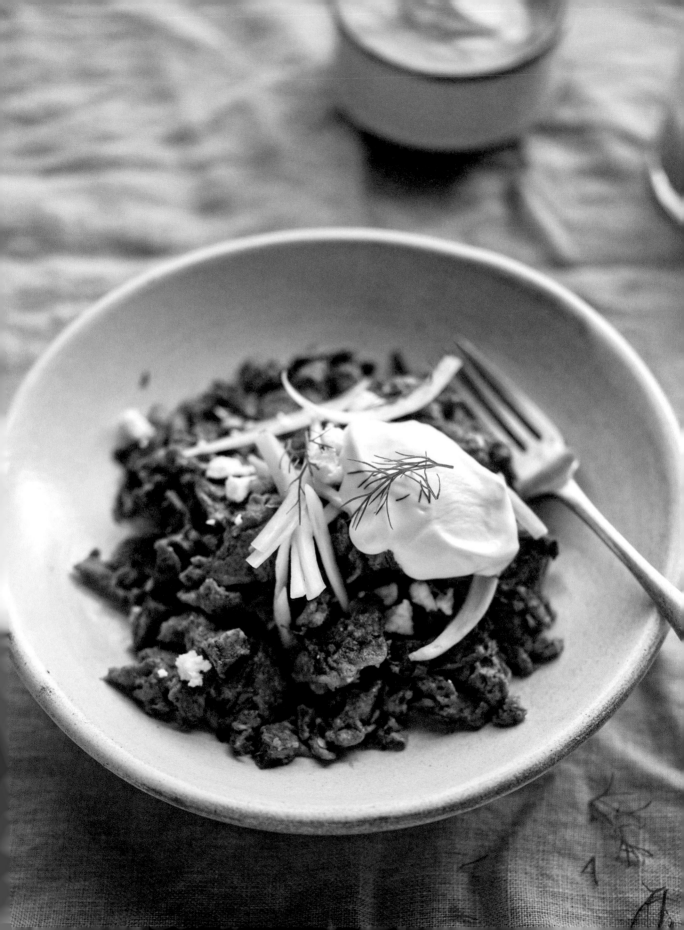

# EGGY MUFFINS
## WITH TURKEY RASHERS, GARLIC AND PARSLEY

I love these so much! They're filling and packed with protein, which is awesome as they will keep you that bit fuller for longer. The beauty of these is that you can change up the combinations as much as you like, as they are so versatile. You can make these in advance and have them stashed in the fridge, ready for breakfast or lunch the next day. A vegetarian version that I adore is roasted red pepper and feta cheese. Gorgeous!

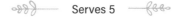 Serves 5

olive oil

6 turkey rashers, finely chopped

3 garlic cloves, finely chopped, or 2 tsp garlic purée

10 eggs

salt and black pepper

5g fresh curly parsley, chopped

low-calorie cooking spray

coleslaw, to serve

Preheat your oven to 190°C.

Heat some olive oil in a frying pan. Add the turkey rashers and garlic and gently fry until the rashers are cooked through, then set aside to cool.

Whisk all the eggs in a large bowl and season well (I love seasoning mine with plenty of black pepper), then stir in the turkey rashers and garlic along with the parsley.

Spray 10 holes of a non-stick muffin tray with low-calorie cooking spray. Use your hands to make sure everything is well greased. Divide the egg mixture evenly between the 10 holes.

Pop into the preheated oven and bake for 18 minutes. Crack over some black pepper and serve with some coleslaw.

**Nutritional Information**

|  | Per Serving |
| --- | --- |
| Calories | 249kcal |
| Protein | 25g |
| Carbohydrates | 3.5g |
| Fat | 15g |
| Gluten Free | ✔ |

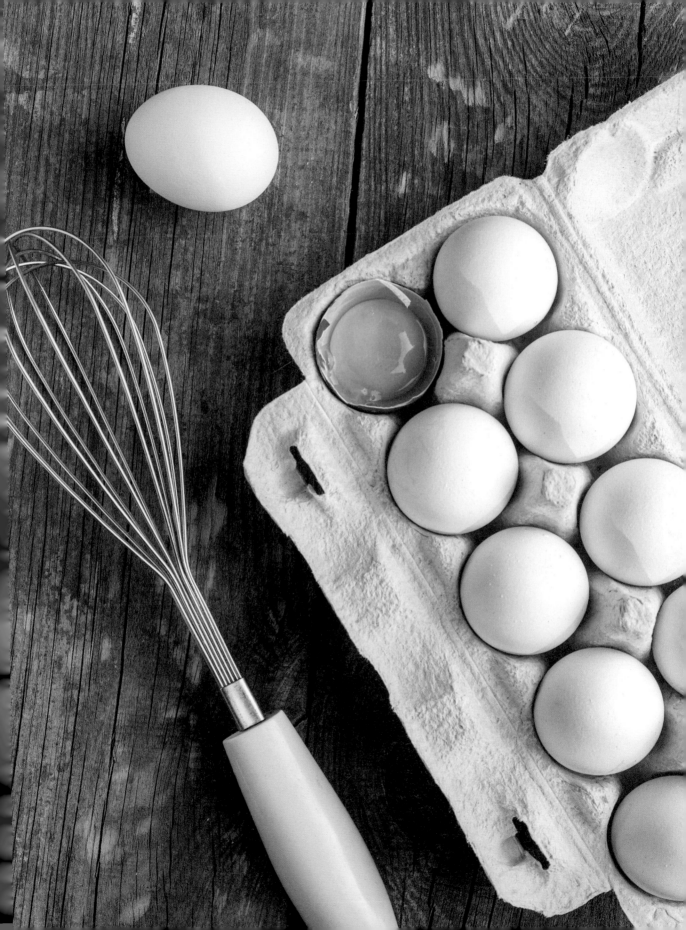

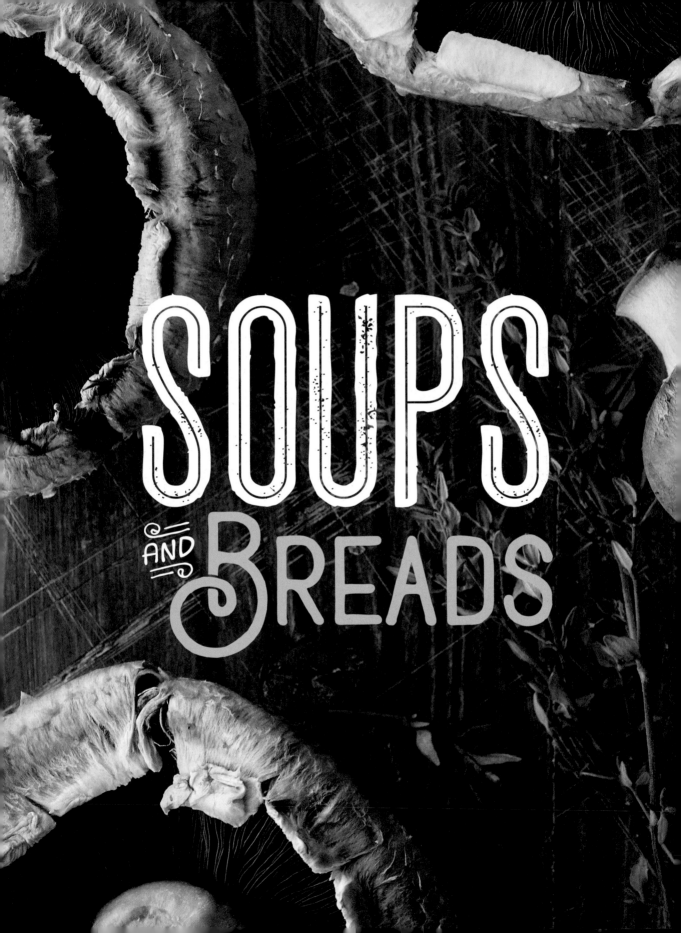

# SOUPS
## AND BREADS

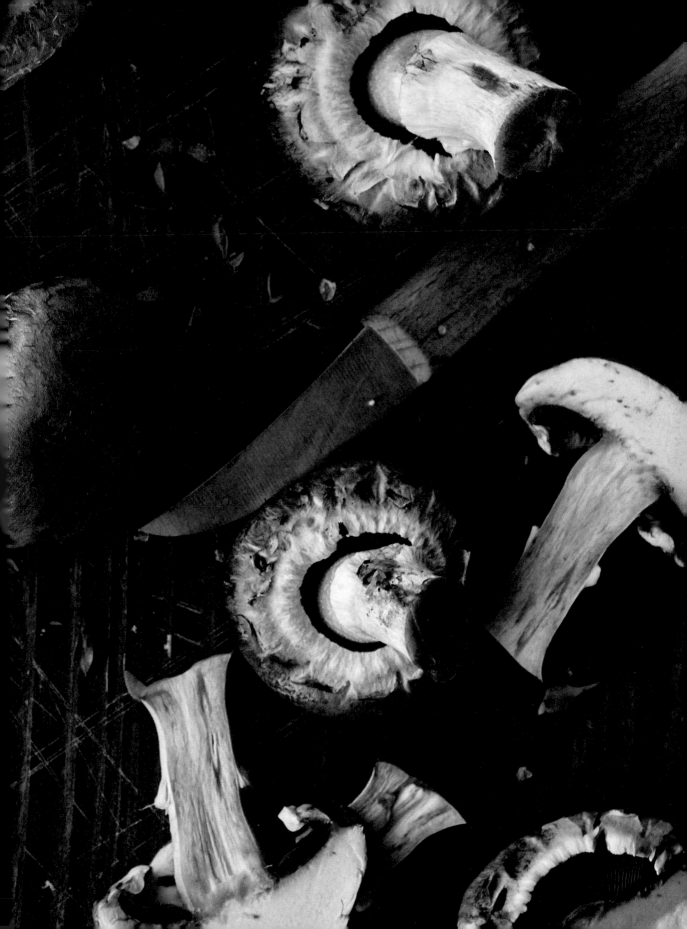

# CHEESE AND ONION WHITE SODA BREAD

Bread is always best eaten on the day that you make it, but if you have it within the next two days, you can always toast it. You can also freeze the slices, then thaw and toast them too.

Makes 12 slices

450g plain flour, plus extra
    for dusting
1 tsp bread soda
    (bicarbonate of soda is
    the same thing)
1 tsp salt
2 medium white onions,
    finely diced
100g light Cheddar cheese,
    grated
350ml buttermilk

Preheat your oven to 220°C. Lightly flour a baking tray. Sieve your flour, bread soda and salt into a large bowl and stir to combine, then add your raw onion and grated cheese and mix together.

Pour in the buttermilk, then using your hand with a claw-like movement, mix it in. Once it's combined into a dough and leaving the sides of the bowl, pop it out on a lightly floured surface and gently shape into a round. Place on the floured tray and make a cross in the middle of the loaf about 2.5cm deep.

Bake in the preheated oven at 220°C for 15 minutes. Reduce the oven temperature to 200°C and bake for 25 more minutes, then turn your bread upside down and bake in the oven for 5 minutes.

Allow to cool on a wire rack, then cut into 12 slices.

**Nutritional Information**

|  | Per Serving |
|---|---|
| Calories | 185kcal |
| Protein | 7g |
| Carbohydrates | 33g |
| Fat | 3g |
| Vegetarian | ✔ |

# BROWN SODA BREAD

You can't beat homemade brown soda bread, from the smell wafting around the house when it's baking to the sheer deliciousness of a slice with a cup of tea. The beauty of Irish brown soda bread is that you need very few ingredients and very little skill to produce an amazing product. Always use a good-quality brown flour, as this will give the bread a slightly nutty texture. The reason for the cross on the top is to let the fairies out!

— Makes 12 slices —

Preheat your oven to 200°C. Lightly dust a baking tray with a little plain flour.

Combine all your dry ingredients in a bowl, then rub in the butter with your fingertips until it's nearly like a crumble.

Pour in the buttermilk, then using your hand with a claw-like movement, mix it in. Once it's combined into a dough and leaving the sides of the bowl, pop it out on a lightly floured surface and gently shape into a round. Place on the floured tray and make a cross in the middle of the loaf about 2.5cm deep.

Bake in the preheated oven for 45 minutes, then turn the bread upside down and bake for another 10 minutes.

Allow to cool on a wire rack, then cut into 12 slices.

265g plain flour,
    plus extra for dusting
265g wholemeal flour
1 tsp bread soda
    (bicarbonate of soda
    is the same thing)
1 tsp salt
30g butter
400ml buttermilk

**Nutritional Information**

|  | Per Serving |
| --- | --- |
| Calories | 180kcal |
| Protein | 6g |
| Carbohydrates | 32g |
| Fat | 3g |
| Vegetarian | ✔ |

# PORRIDGE BREAD

The classic porridge bread. This is full of fibre and is delicious with some of the berry, cinnamon and orange compote on page 205.

Makes 10 slices

500g low-fat natural
 yoghurt
2 tsp bread soda
 (bicarbonate of soda
 is the same thing)
1 tsp salt
350g porridge oats
1 egg, beaten
1 tbsp low-fat milk

Preheat your oven to 180°C. Line a 2lb loaf tin with non-stick baking paper.

Mix your yoghurt, bread soda and salt in a large bowl, then mix in the oats. Make a well in the centre, then add your egg and milk. Mix gently until everything is combined, then scrape into the lined loaf tin and level the top.

Pop in the preheated oven for 45 minutes. Remove the loaf from the tin, put it directly on the oven rack and bake in the oven for 15 more minutes.

Allow to cool on a wire rack, then cut into 10 slices.

**Nutritional Information**

|  | Per Serving |
| --- | --- |
| Calories | 211kcal |
| Protein | 7g |
| Carbohydrates | 26g |
| Fat | 8g |
| Vegetarian | ✔ |

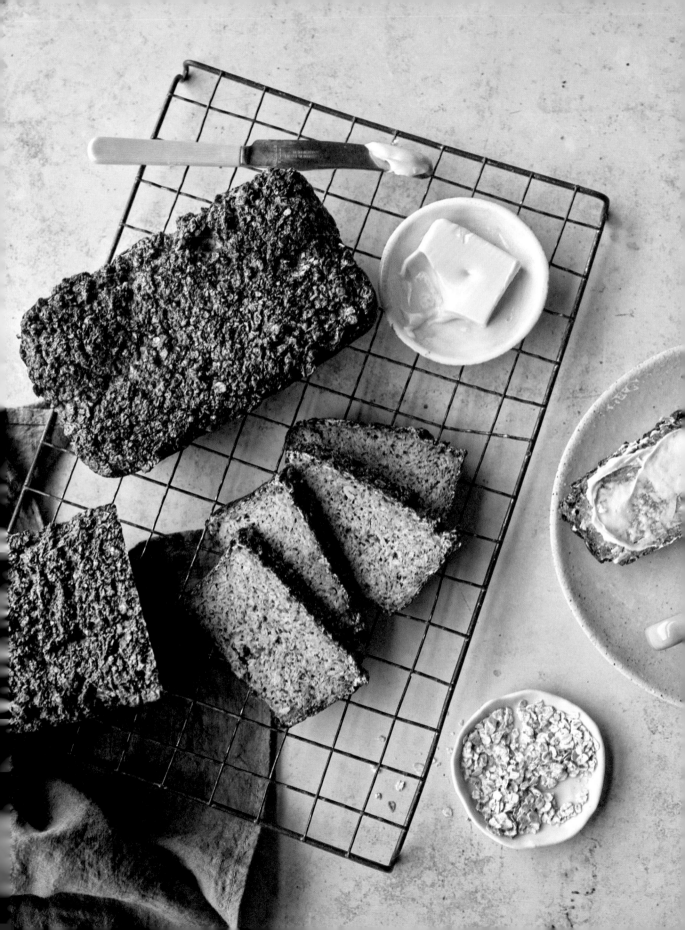

# VEGAN BROWN SODA BREAD

This is so delicious and you would be hard pushed to taste the difference between this and regular brown soda bread! I use oat milk as it's naturally sweeter and slightly thicker than other plant-based milks. Each slice is low in calories and a lovely snack option to have.

*Makes 10 slices*

200g plain flour, plus extra for dusting

150g wholemeal flour

1 tsp bread soda (bicarbonate of soda is the same thing)

1 tsp salt

200ml oat milk

1 medium lemon, juiced

Preheat your oven to 200°C. Lightly dust a baking tray with a little plain flour.

Combine all your dry ingredients in a bowl and make a well in the centre.

Mix your oat milk and lemon juice together in a jug, then pour it into the dry ingredients. Using your hand with a claw-like movement, mix it in. Once it's combined into a dough and leaving the sides of the bowl, pop it out on a lightly floured surface and gently shape into a round. Place on the floured tray and make a cross in the middle of the loaf about 2.5cm deep.

Bake in the preheated oven for 30 minutes, then turn the bread upside down and bake for another 10 minutes.

Allow to cool on a wire rack, then cut into 10 slices.

**Nutritional Information**

|  | Per Serving |
| --- | --- |
| Calories | 134kcal |
| Protein | 3.5g |
| Carbohydrates | 27g |
| Fat | 1g |
| Vegetarian | ✔ |

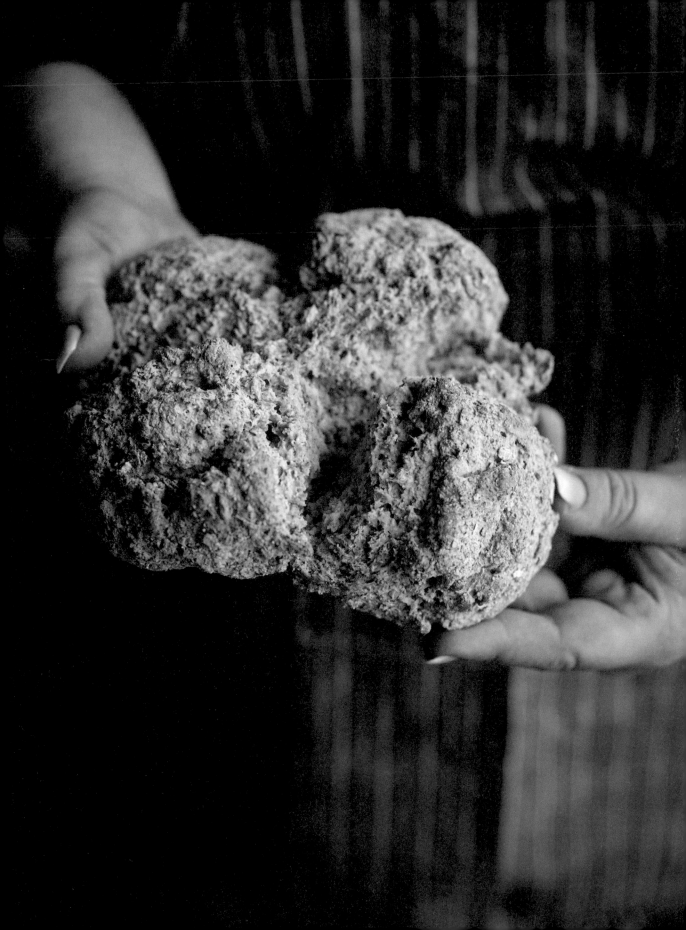

# COCONUT BREAD

This can be a dangerous one, as it's just so delicious. Once it's cooled,
make sure you slice it up and pop it into the freezer ASAP
so that you won't eat it all in one day!

—∂∂♪— Makes 15 slices —ᖶᖳᖳ—

low-calorie cooking spray, for
    greasing
125g caster sugar
130ml buttermilk
75ml olive oil
4 eggs
2 tsp vanilla extract
385g plain flour
125g desiccated coconut
100g chopped walnuts
1 tsp baking powder
1 tsp bread soda (bicarbonate
    of soda is the same thing)
½ tsp salt

Preheat your oven to 180°C. Grease 2 x 1lb loaf tins with low-calorie cooking spray.

Put your sugar, buttermilk, oil, eggs and vanilla in a large bowl and whisk together. Add your flour, coconut, walnuts, baking powder, bread soda and salt and mix again until well combined.

Pour into your two greased tins and level the tops. Bake in the preheated oven for 1 hour, then allow to cool on a wire rack.

Make sure you cut the two loaves into 15 slices in total to keep the calorie count down.

**Nutritional Information**

|  | Per Serving |
| --- | --- |
| Calories | 295kcal |
| Protein | 6g |
| Carbohydrates | 31g |
| Fat | 16g |
| Vegetarian | ✔ |

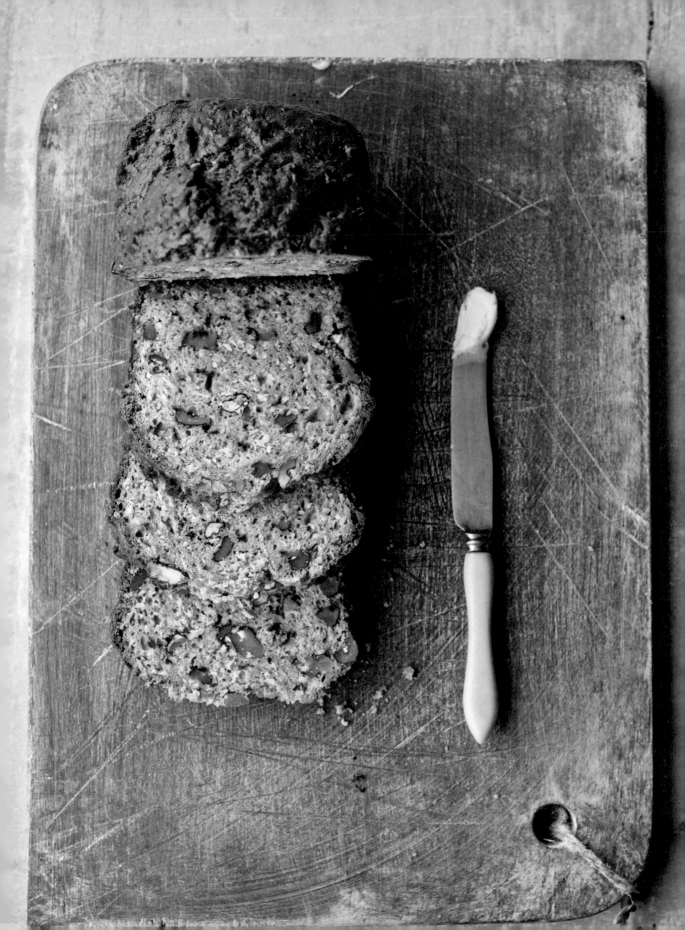

# MEDITERRANEAN-STYLE ROASTED RED PEPPER SOUP

For years in the restaurant, this was one of my favourite soups and I would always garnish it with pesto. The key is to roast most of your vegetables here to enhance the flavour. I use red onion in my mirepoix for that delicious sweet flavour. A little bit of feta crumbled on top is a nice optional extra.

Serves 4

3 red peppers, chopped

2 red onions, chopped

3 garlic cloves, chopped

1 tsp coriander seeds or ground coriander

salt and black pepper

2 tbsp olive oil, plus extra for cooking

2 celery sticks

1 x 400g tin of chopped tomatoes

1 vegetable stock cube

300ml boiling water

fresh basil leaves, to garnish

vegan brown soda bread (page 102), to serve

Preheat your oven to 180°C.

Put your peppers, onions, garlic and coriander on a large baking tray and season with salt and pepper, then drizzle with the 2 tablespoons of olive oil and toss to coat. Roast in the preheated oven for 30 minutes, until the veg are soft and caramelised.

Meanwhile, heat a large pot and add a splash of olive oil. Add the celery and gently sauté until softened, then add your chopped tomatoes and simmer for 10 minutes to draw out their sweetness.

Dissolve the stock cube in the hot water, then pour into the tomato mixture, stirring to combine. Simmer for 10 minutes.

Add your roasted vegetables to the pot, then using a hand-held blender, blitz until creamy and smooth. Ladle into warmed bowls and garnish with a few fresh basil leaves and cracked black pepper. Serve with a slice of vegan brown soda bread. This will last for three days in your fridge once chilled.

## Nutritional Information

| | Per Serving |
|---|---|
| Calories | 170kcal |
| Protein | 4g |
| Carbohydrates | 12g |
| Fat | 12g |
| Vegetarian | ✔ |

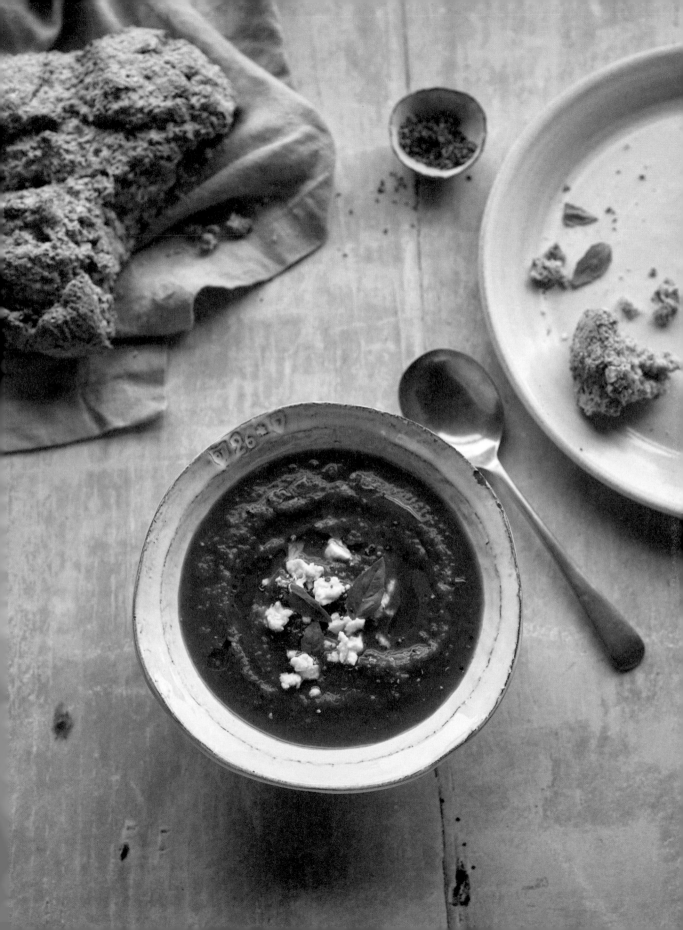

# MUSHROOM SOUP WITH PARSLEY

My favourite soup is mushroom and my favourite combination is mushroom and garlic, so this is a winner for me! My sister Ellen taught me this recipe and I make it for my family every Christmas Day. To reduce the calories, you could swap light coconut milk for the cream. It seems like a lot of mushrooms, but trust me, they're made up of a lot of water so they shrink a lot when cooked.

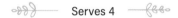 Serves 4

olive oil

1 white onion, chopped

4 celery sticks, chopped

2 large garlic cloves, chopped

500g button mushrooms, sliced

200g flat mushrooms, sliced

800ml boiling water

2 vegetable stock cubes

100ml light cream, plus extra
   to garnish

½ lemon, juiced

salt and black pepper

chopped fresh flat-leaf parsley, to
   garnish

Heat a large heavy-based pot and add some oil. Add the onion, celery and garlic – this is your mirepoix, which is your flavour base. Once these are softened, add your mushrooms and cook for 5 minutes. Take out a few of the button mushroom slices for garnish and set aside.

Pour in your water and stock cubes, stirring to dissolve the stock cubes, and simmer for 10 minutes. Add your cream and simmer for a further 5 minutes, then stir in the lemon juice and season well with salt and pepper. Blitz with a hand-held blender until smooth.

Ladle into warmed bowls and garnish with the cream, reserved mushroom slices and the chopped fresh parsley. This will last for three days in your fridge once chilled.

## Nutritional Information

|  | Per Serving |
| --- | --- |
| Calories | 155kcal |
| Protein | 9g |
| Carbohydrates | 16g |
| Fat | 6g |
| Vegetarian | ✔ |

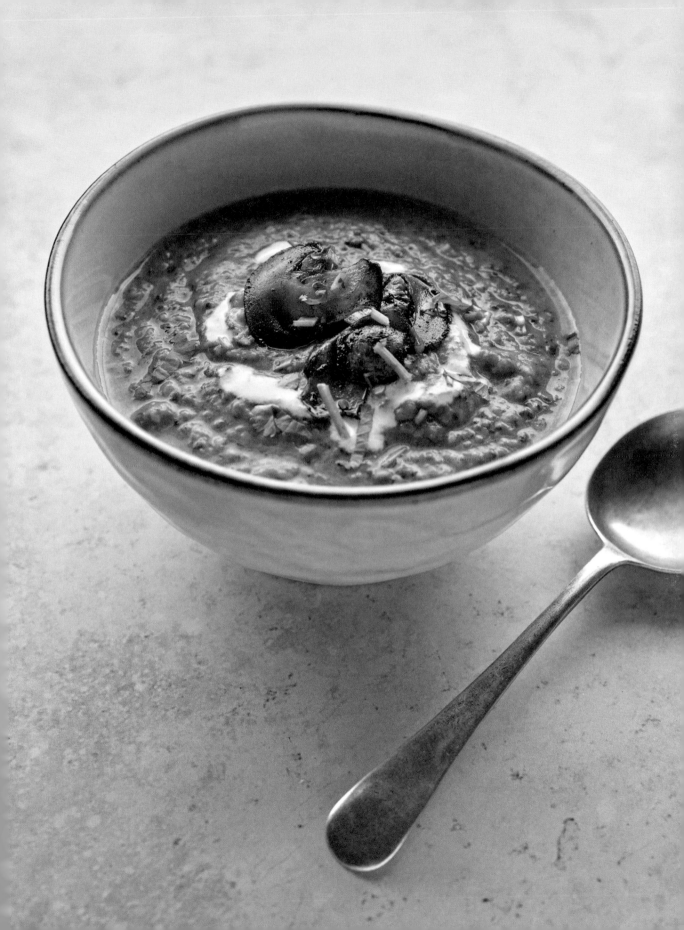

# CHICKEN CURRY SOUP

This is a bowl of love. If you have leftover roast chicken (page 130), this is the perfect way to use it up. In the restaurant I used a food processor to blend up the vegetables, but if you don't have one, a regular box grater will do the same job. If you're like me and like spicy food, you can add an extra chilli for heat. This is packed with protein and you could swap brown rice for the basmati if you'd like to pack in some extra fibre.

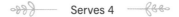 Serves 4

400g cooked chicken or raw chicken breast
olive oil
1 tbsp mild curry powder
1 tsp cumin seeds
1 tsp ground coriander
1 tsp wholegrain mustard
2 white onions, grated
2 carrots, grated
2 parsnips, grated
3 garlic cloves, grated
1 fresh red chilli, deseeded and finely diced
2.5cm piece of fresh ginger, peeled and
    grated
2 chicken stock cubes
1 litre boiling water
50g basmati rice (uncooked weight)
salt and black pepper
1 lime, cut into wedges, to serve
fresh coriander leaves, to garnish

If you have leftover roast chicken, then simply run your knife through it to shred it. If you're cooking it from scratch, pop your chicken breast in a pan of cold water and bring to the boil, then reduce the heat and simmer for 30 minutes. Remove from the pan and run under cold water, then shred.

Heat a large heavy-based casserole or pot and add some oil. Add your curry powder, cumin seeds, coriander and mustard. Fry for 1 minute, until you can smell the spices.

Add your onions, carrots, parsnips, garlic, chilli and ginger. Pour in a splash of water and pop a lid on top, as this will create steam and help to cook your vegetables faster. Cook until softened.

Dissolve the stock cubes in the hot water, then pour it into the pot along with the shredded chicken and the rice. Cover the pot and simmer for 20 minutes so that the rice cooks and absorbs all the flavours. Season with salt and pepper.

To serve, ladle into warmed bowls with lime wedges and garnish with fresh coriander leaves. This will last for three days in your fridge once chilled.

## Nutritional Information

| | Per Serving |
|---|---|
| Calories | 376kcal |
| Protein | 25g |
| Carbohydrates | 33g |
| Fat | 16g |

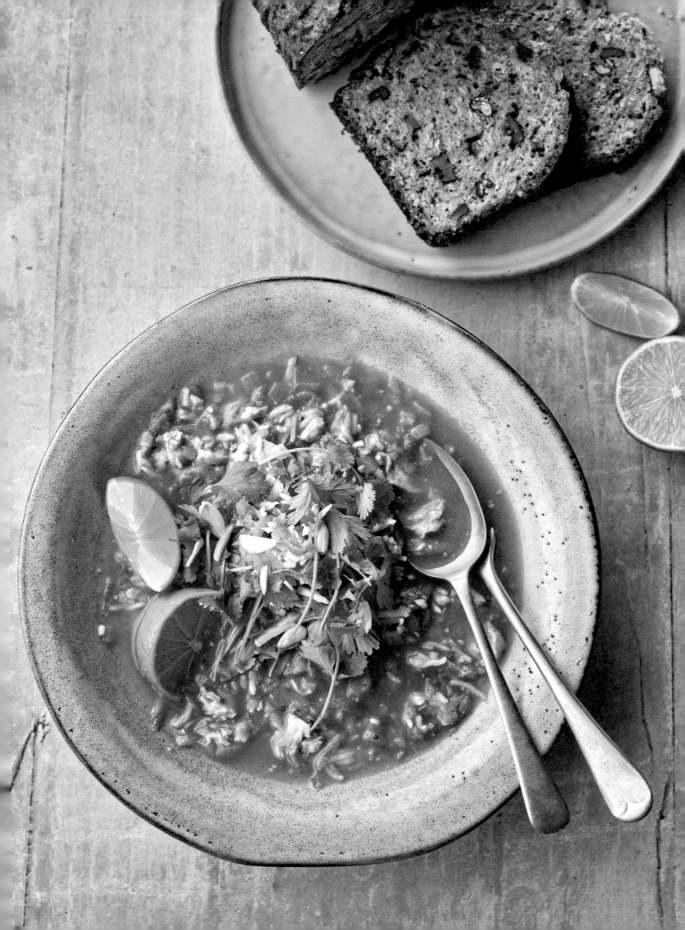

# BUTTER BEAN SOUP

This will warm you up and fill you with the feeling of goodness. There's a Mediterranean feel to the dish. I always use tinned beans as they are less hassle than the dried version and much quicker to cook.

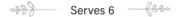 Serves 6

low-calorie cooking spray

1 red onion, diced

4 celery sticks, diced

3 garlic cloves, chopped

2 carrots, diced

2 red peppers, diced

1 courgette, diced

1 tsp paprika

1 tsp chilli powder

salt and black pepper

1 x 500g carton of passata

1 x 400g tin of chopped tomatoes

400ml water

2 vegetable stock cubes

2 bay leaves

1 tbsp light soy sauce

2 x 400g tins of butter beans, drained and rinsed

6 cubes of frozen kale or spinach

spring onions, thinly sliced, to garnish

Heat a large pot and add some low-calorie spray. Add your onion, celery and garlic and sauté until softened. Add your carrots, peppers, courgette, paprika, chilli powder and some salt and pepper and cook for 1 minute.

Pour in your passata, chopped tomatoes, water, stock cubes, bay leaves and soy sauce and bring to the boil. Add your butter beans, then reduce the heat and simmer for 30 minutes to allow the flavours to marry. Add your frozen kale and simmer for 5 minutes, then season to taste with salt and pepper.

To serve, ladle into warmed bowls and garnish with spring onions. This will last for three days in your fridge once chilled.

**Nutritional Information**

|  | Per Serving |
| --- | --- |
| Calories | 176kcal |
| Protein | 8g |
| Carbohydrates | 27g |
| Fat | 5g |
| Vegetarian | ✔ |

# LIGHTLY SPICED PUMPKIN SOUP

At Halloween we're all carving pumpkins but are often at a loss for what to do with the leftovers. Well, here you go! This is like a hug in a bowl and is gorgeous for lunch on a cold day. The reason why there's two styles of cooking here (roasting and boiling) is because you're enhancing the flavour of the pumpkin and giving it a creamy texture.

Serves 6

Preheat your oven to 180°C.

Chop your pumpkin into small chunks, including the skin and seeds. Place on a large baking tray with your chilli flakes, cumin, coriander, salt and pepper and olive oil. Use your hands to toss the pumpkin in the spices and olive oil so that everything gets evenly coated. Place in the preheated oven for 1 hour to roast and caramelise.

Meanwhile, heat a large pot and add a drop of olive oil.

Add your onions, carrot and garlic and gently sauté until softened. Dissolve the stock cubes in the hot water, then pour into the pot. Leave to simmer for 20 minutes.

Combine your roasted pumpkin with your stock mixture and blitz with a hand-held blender until creamy and smooth. Up to this point the soup is vegan, but if you would like to add the cream, do so now.

To serve, ladle into warmed bowls. This will last for three days in your fridge once chilled.

1 medium pumpkin
 (about 1.2kg)
2 tsp chilli flakes
2 tsp ground cumin
2 tsp ground coriander
salt and black pepper
100ml olive oil, plus extra for
 cooking
2 white onions, finely
 chopped
1 carrot, finely chopped
3 garlic cloves, finely
 chopped
2 vegetable stock cubes
1 litre boiling water
50ml light cream (optional)

## Nutritional Information

|  | Per Serving |
| --- | --- |
| Calories | 302kcal |
| Protein | 7g |
| Carbohydrates | 23g |
| Fat | 19g |
| Vegetarian | ✔ |

# PEA, BACON AND MINT SOUP

This is so simple and easy to make. Adding the spinach at the end will give your soup a burst of green colour and give your body a burst of vitamin D and nutrients! This is a very summery soup, as it's light yet filling at the same time. I use frozen petit pois as they are smaller and sweeter. The saltiness and smokiness from the bacon adds that extra punch. Delicious!

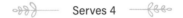

Serves 4

400g frozen petit pois

olive oil

1 white onion, diced

2 garlic cloves, chopped

50g smoked streaky bacon, chopped

2 vegetable stock cubes

400ml boiling water

400g spinach (fresh or frozen)

100ml light cream, plus extra to garnish

1 lemon, juiced

salt and black pepper

10g fresh mint leaves, plus extra to garnish

Bring a small pot of water to the boil, then add your frozen peas. As soon as the water comes back to the boil, strain the peas and run them under cold water. (This method of cooking is called blanching and it helps to keep the peas' bright green colour.)

Heat a large pot and add some olive oil. Add your onion, garlic and bacon and gently sauté until the onion has softened.

Dissolve the stock cubes in the hot water, then pour into the pot and simmer for 5 minutes. Add your blanched peas and spinach and simmer for 5 minutes, then add your cream, lemon juice and mint and simmer for 3 minutes. Blitz with a hand-held blender until smooth, then season with salt and pepper.

To serve, ladle into warmed bowls and garnish with a little cream and a few fresh mint leaves. This will last for three days in your fridge once chilled.

**Nutritional Information**

|  | Per Serving |
|---|---|
| Calories | 209kcal |
| Protein | 13g |
| Carbohydrates | 14g |
| Fat | 11g |

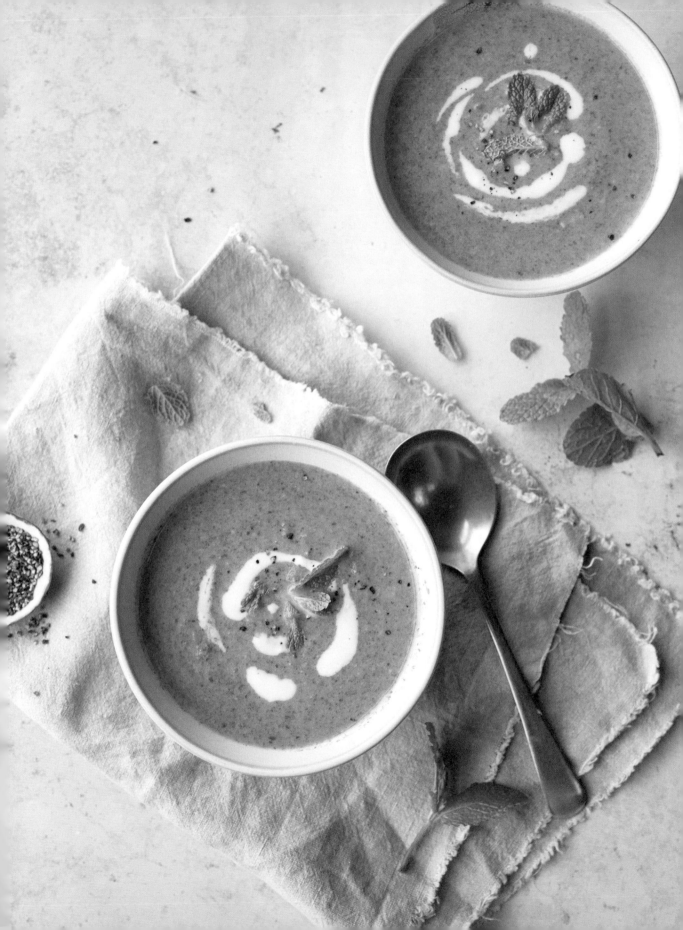

# MEXICAN SHRIMP SOUP

I love this soup because it's like a fancy hot prawn cocktail. It's a winner because shrimps are available in most freezer aisles and it's so simple and fast to make. It's also high in protein as soups go.

Serves 4

olive oil

1 red onion, finely diced

1 carrot, grated

1 celery stick, finely diced

3 garlic cloves, finely chopped

1 fresh green chilli, deseeded and finely chopped

1 tsp chilli flakes

1 tsp ground cumin

1 tsp smoked paprika (regular paprika is okay too)

1 tsp dried oregano

1 x 400g tin of chopped tomatoes

250g sweet potatoes, peeled and diced

1 tbsp tomato purée

200g frozen shrimp (run under cold water to defrost)

200ml water

1 small ripe avocado

1 bunch of fresh coriander, chopped

1 fresh red chilli, deseeded and thinly sliced, to garnish

1 lime, cut into wedges, to serve

Heat a large pot and add some olive oil. Add your onion, carrot, celery and garlic and sauté until softened. Add your fresh green chilli, chilli flakes, cumin, paprika and oregano and fry for 1 minute.

Add your chopped tomatoes, sweet potatoes and tomato purée and simmer for 20 minutes to allow the potatoes to cook and the flavours to marry.

Add your shrimp and water and simmer for 4 minutes. Don't cook the shrimp for too long or they will become tiny and tough.

Mash your avocado and coriander together in a bowl.

To serve, ladle into warmed bowls with a dollop of your avocado mixture and red chilli slices on top and lime wedges on the side.

### Nutritional Information

| | Per Serving |
|---|---|
| Calories | 239kcal |
| Protein | 14g |
| Carbohydrates | 25g |
| Fat | 9g |
| Gluten Free | ✔ |

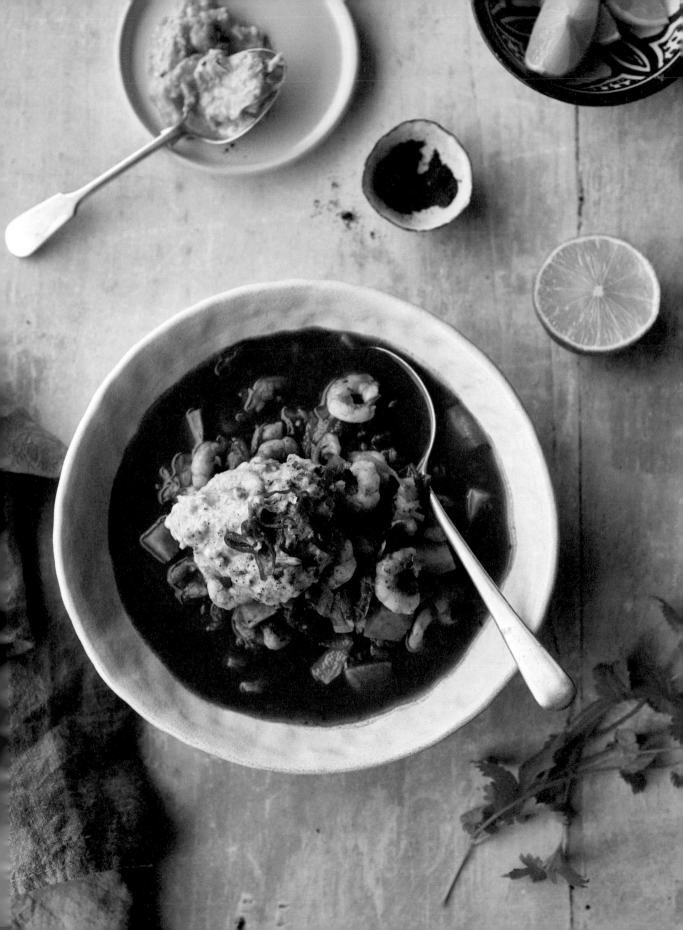

# SEAFOOD CHOWDER

I love chowder so much. When I can get fresh dill, I always pick it up and make some chowder. If you can't source dill, flat-leaf parsley and chives are also amazing herbs with chowder. This is so simple to make and the more varieties of fish you have, the better. If you're making a big pot, try to get some smoked haddock in the mix – you'll love it. Chowder is filling so it's an ideal lunch, but if you have it with bread it's a healthy dinner with a good portion of protein per serving.

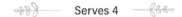 Serves 4

olive oil

1 white onion, diced

1 leek, thinly sliced

2 garlic cloves, chopped

15g plain flour

3 fish or vegetable stock cubes

500ml boiling water

500ml low-fat milk

2 large potatoes, diced small

1/2 red pepper, thinly sliced

100g smoked salmon

100g white fish (cod, hake, pollock or all three)

50g frozen shrimp

salt and white pepper

1 bunch of fresh dill, chopped (reserve some for garnish)

brown soda bread (page 99), to serve

Heat a large saucepan and add some olive oil. Add your onion, leek and garlic and sauté until softened. Stir in your flour and cook for 1 more minute.

Dissolve your stock cubes in the hot water, then add to the saucepan along with the milk, stirring constantly with a whisk to get rid of any flour lumps.

Add your potatoes and pepper and simmer for 10 minutes, then add your smoked salmon and white fish and simmer for another 10 minutes.

Add your shrimp and simmer for 5 minutes. Don't cook these for too long or they will become tough and rubbery. Season with salt and white pepper and stir in your dill.

Ladle into warmed bowls and garnish with a little extra dill. Serve straight away with some yummy brown soda bread on the side.

## Nutritional Information

|  | Per Serving |
| --- | --- |
| Calories | 303kcal |
| Protein | 20g |
| Carbohydrates | 34g |
| Fat | 9g |

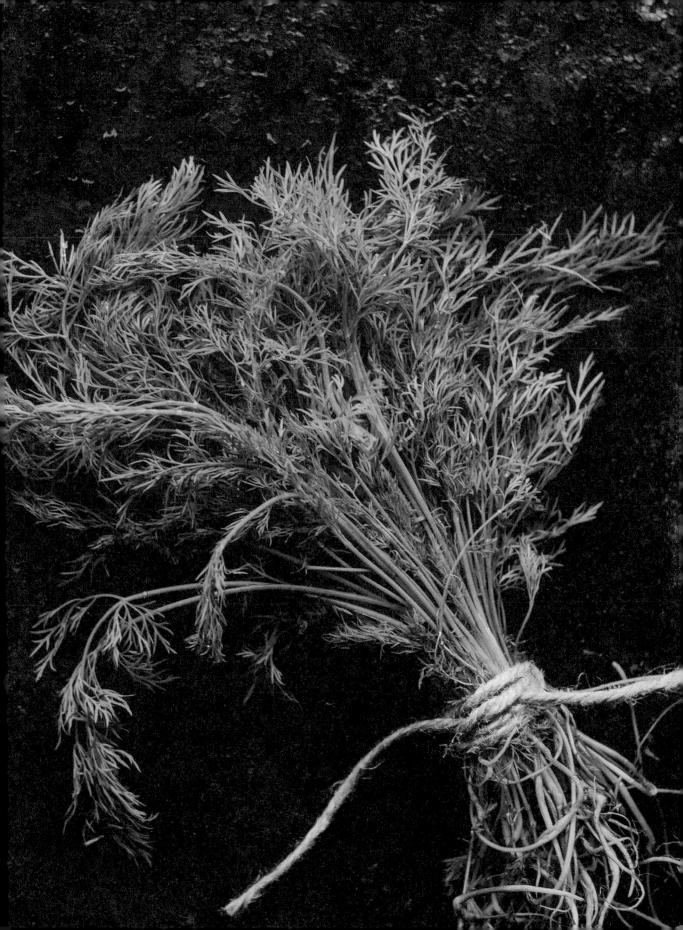

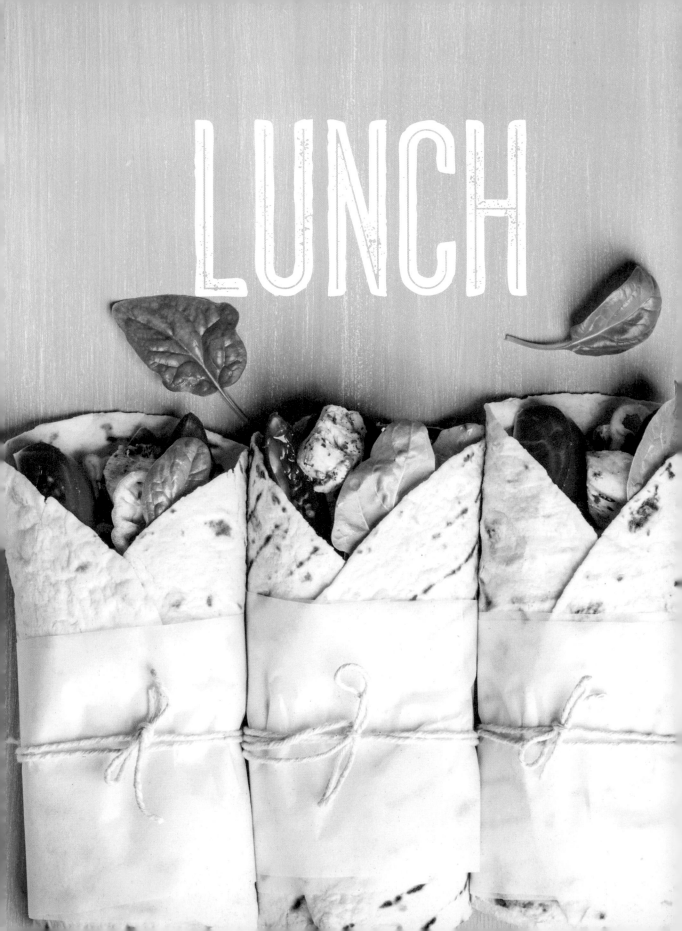

# LUNCH

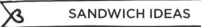

## SANDWICH IDEAS

Lunch can sometimes be overwhelming, so here are some of my mix-and-match
ideas for handy go-to sambos. I love toasted sandwiches too, so you can always do that to change it up!

| Bread<br>**Pick one and toast** | Spread<br>**Pick one** | Protein<br>**Pick one** | Cheese<br>**Pick one** | Extra<br>**As many as you like to bulk up your sandwich** |
|---|---|---|---|---|
| Wrap | Lighter-than-light mayonnaise | Chicken breast | Feta | Onion |
| Brown soda bread | | Turkey breast | Cheddar | Tomato |
| Brown bread | Pesto | Lean ham | Goats cheese | Cucumber |
| Ciabatta | Hummus | Lean beef | Brie | Peppers |
| Pitta bread | Sriracha | Coronation chicken | | Rocket |
| Bagel | | Eggs | | Cos lettuce |
| | | Tuna and sweetcorn | | Spinach |
| | | Tinned sardines | | Basil |

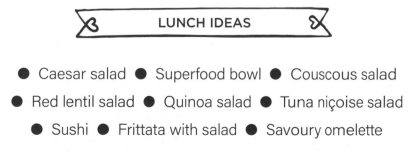

## LUNCH IDEAS

● Caesar salad ● Superfood bowl ● Couscous salad
● Red lentil salad ● Quinoa salad ● Tuna niçoise salad
● Sushi ● Frittata with salad ● Savoury omelette

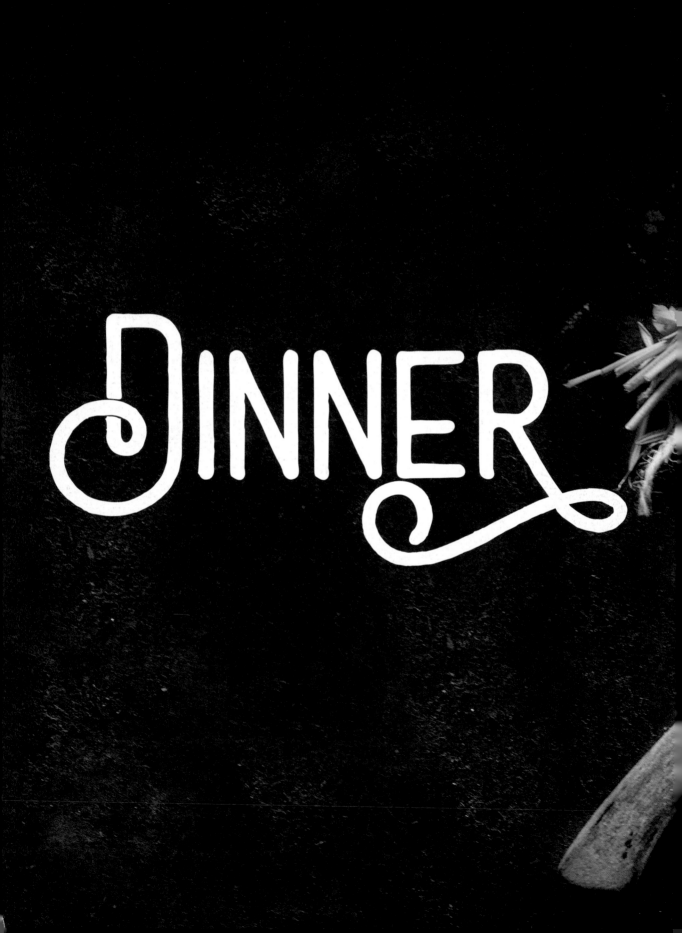

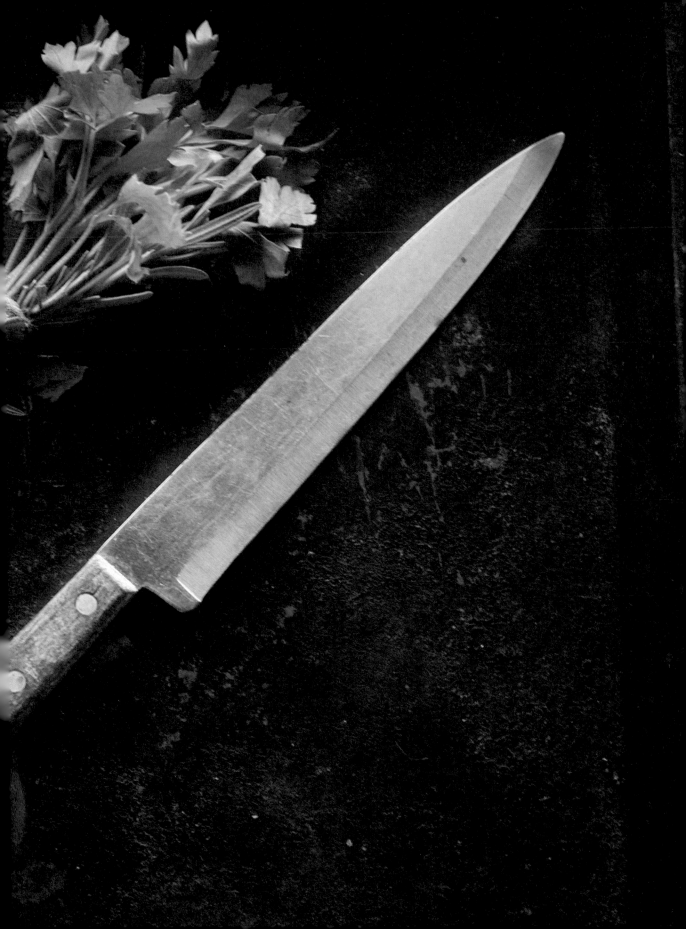

# BEEF SATAY
## WITH SHREDDED CARROT

An amazing fake-away that reheats very well. I personally use fillet of beef, as it's much more tender and juicy. Avoid stewing beef, as it won't be cooking for long enough to tenderise it. Make sure that you stir your sauce frequently, as it does have a tendency to stick.

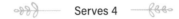 Serves 4

olive oil

400g fillet steak, cut into thin strips

5 small or 3 large carrots, grated

4 spring onions, thinly sliced

1 red pepper, thinly sliced

3 garlic cloves, finely chopped

1 small chilli, deseeded and diced

45g 100% nuts peanut butter

1 x 400ml tin of low-fat coconut milk

40ml light soy sauce

fresh coriander leaves, to garnish

roasted peanuts, to garnish

boiled basmati rice or noodles, to serve

Heat a large saucepan and add some oil. Add your steak, carrots, spring onions, pepper, garlic and chilli and sauté for a few minutes.

Stir in your peanut butter, coconut milk and soy sauce and bring to the boil, then lower the heat and simmer for 15 minutes, until the sauce has reduced and thickened slightly.

Garnish with fresh coriander leaves and a few roasted peanuts and serve with basmati rice or noodles.

**Nutritional Information**

|  | Per Serving |
|---|---|
| Calories | 390kcal |
| Protein | 28g |
| Carbohydrates | 19g |
| Fat | 22g |
| Gluten Free | ✔ |

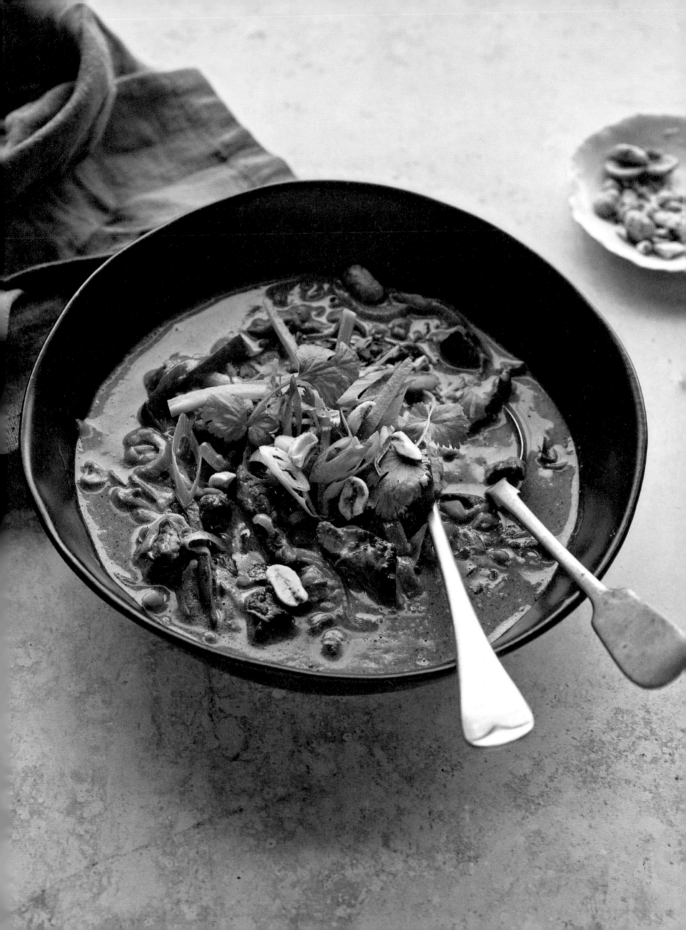

# BEEF AND MUSHROOM QUESADILLAS

The key to quesadillas is nice moist fillings and a crisp tortilla. An amazing lunch or dinner, these are packed with protein. These are so good with some reduced-fat sour cream on the side, but note that adding that would change your macros.

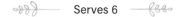 Serves 6

low-calorie cooking spray

250g stir-fry beef

1 red onion, diced

4 button mushrooms, sliced

2 garlic cloves, finely chopped

2 fresh red chillies, deseeded and diced

salt and black pepper

1 tsp chilli powder

1 x 400g tin of chickpeas, drained and rinsed

400g passata

1 tsp chopped fresh mint

1 tsp chopped fresh coriander

6 brown tortilla wraps

280g light red Cheddar cheese, grated

fresh coriander leaves, to garnish

1 lime, cut into wedges, to garnish

guacamole (page 173), to serve

rocket salad, to serve

Heat a saucepan and add some low-calorie cooking spray. Add your beef, onion, mushrooms, garlic, fresh red chillies and some salt and pepper and cook until the onion has softened and the beef has browned. Add your chilli powder and cook for 1 minute.

Add your chickpeas and passata and simmer for 20 minutes, until the sauce has reduced and thickened. Transfer the mixture to a bowl and stir in your mint and coriander.

Heat a large frying pan and add some low-calorie spray. Add one tortilla wrap and spoon in one-third of the beef mixture. Scatter over one-third of the grated cheese and place another wrap on top. Leave crisp up for 3 minutes and flip over with a spatula or a fish slice. Cook for 3 minutes. Repeat with the remaining tortilla wraps, filling and cheese.

Cut into quarters and garnish with fresh coriander leaves. Serve 2 quarters per person, with lime wedges and some guacamole (page 173) and a rocket salad on the side.

## Nutritional Information

| | Per Serving |
|---|---|
| Calories | 475kcal |
| Protein | 28g |
| Carbohydrates | 54g |
| Fat | 16g |

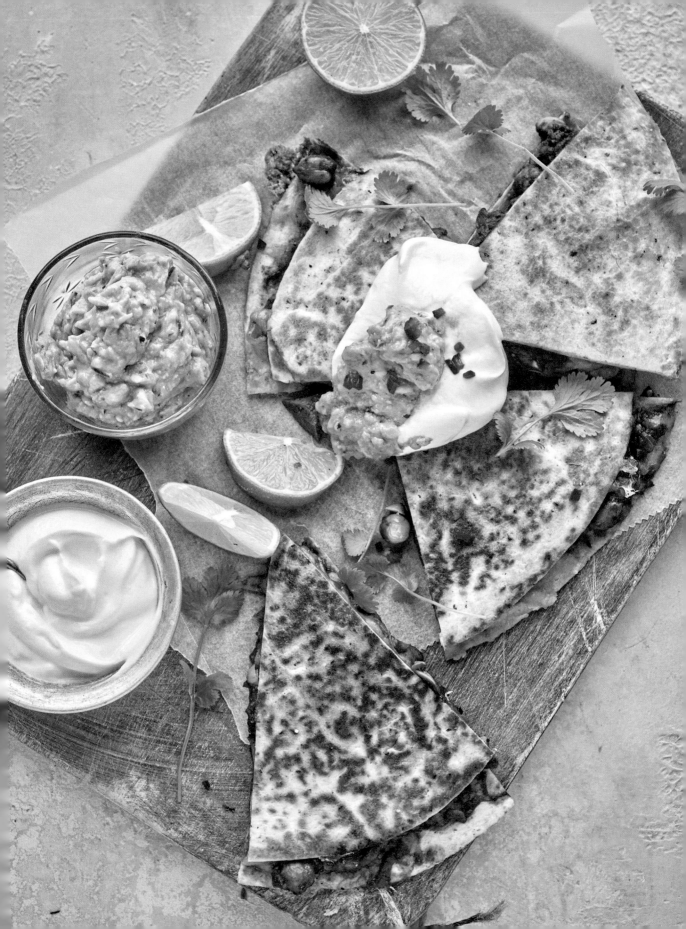

# ROAST BEEF

I think people are afraid of making a roast dinner, but it's actually so simple and not one bit complicated. Once you have a really good cut of beef, some onions and herbs and some time, you are ready to rock! I love sirloin of beef mainly because of the fat, which I know isn't the most ideal cut if you're battling the bulge! So these days I tend to go for a fillet of beef or remove some of the fat off the sirloin beforehand. You can sear it on a hot pan first, but to be honest, I don't bother. What I do instead is roast it in the oven at a really hot temperature for the first 15 minutes to get the crispness going. Housekeeper's cut is always delicious too. Any leftovers can be used for a beef stir-fry or in sandwiches for lunch the next day.

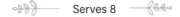 Serves 8

3 white onions, chopped into chunky pieces

4 celery sticks, chopped into chunky pieces

1 carrot, chopped into chunky pieces

5 whole, unpeeled garlic cloves

2kg prime cut of beef, such as sirloin or fillet

cup of water

olive oil

salt and black pepper

5 sprigs of fresh rosemary or thyme, leaves stripped and chopped

hasselback potatoes (page 188), to serve

salsa verde (page 177), to serve

Preheat your oven to 220°C.

Scatter your chunky chopped vegetables and whole garlic cloves in a roasting tray (this is called a trivet) and pop your beef on top, then pour a cup of water into the tray. Rub a little olive oil on top of the beef, then season well with salt and pepper and scatter over the herbs.

Roast in the preheated oven for 15 minutes, then reduce the oven temperature to 180°C and cook for a further 1 hour 30 minutes for a medium roast or 2 hours for well done.

Remove from the oven and leave it to rest for at least 15 minutes before carving.

Serve with hasselback potatoes and salsa verde on the side.

**Nutritional Information**

|  | Per Serving |
| --- | --- |
| Calories | 598kcal |
| Protein | 86g |
| Carbohydrates | 6g |
| Fat | 25g |
| Gluten Free | ✔ |

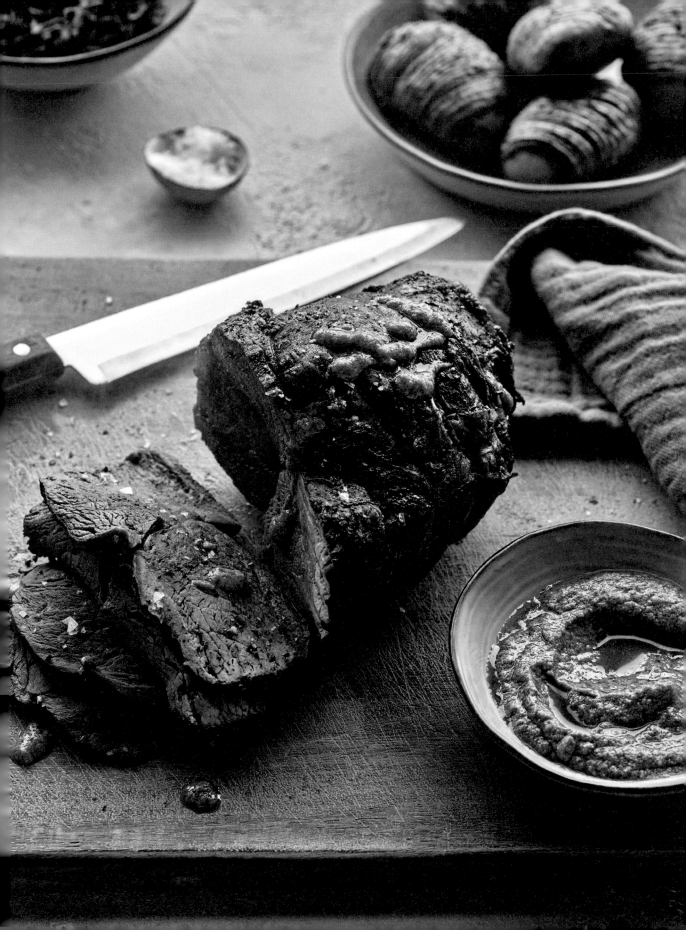

# ROAST CHICKEN

I just love a roast chicken on a Sunday. The key to a good roast chicken is using a trivet of vegetables and a glass of water. As a chef using combi ovens in restaurant kitchens, this is how I create steam in the oven and extra flavour. The perfect roast chicken should have crispy skin on the outside and juicy meat on the inside. The vegetables on the tray can be eaten as part of your dish.

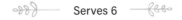 Serves 6

2 white onions, halved or chopped into chunky pieces

2 carrots, chopped into chunky pieces

4 celery sticks, chopped into chunky pieces

4 whole garlic cloves, unpeeled

4 sprigs of fresh thyme, plus extra to garnish

1 x 1.5 kg whole chicken

1 tbsp olive oil

salt and black pepper

100ml cold water

cheesy cauliflower (page 194) and garlic and rosemary mashed potatoes (page 186), to serve

Preheat your oven to 200°C.

Scatter your chunky chopped vegetables, whole garlic cloves and thyme sprigs in a roasting tray (this is the trivet) and pop your chicken on top. Remove the string from around the chicken legs, then rub the olive oil on top of the chicken and season well with salt and pepper. Pour your water around the vegetables.

Roast in the preheated oven for 40 minutes, then reduce the oven temperature to 180°C and cook for 50 minutes more. To check if the chicken is done, pierce the thickest part of the chicken between the leg and the body – if the juices run clear, your chicken is ready.

Leave to rest for 10 minutes before carving and serving. Do not cover it with tin foil, as the water will keep it moist and this way the skin will stay crisp.

**Nutritional Information**

|  | Per Serving |
| --- | --- |
| Calories | 620kcal |
| Protein | 67g |
| Carbohydrates | 10g |
| Fat | 34g |
| Gluten Free | ✔ |

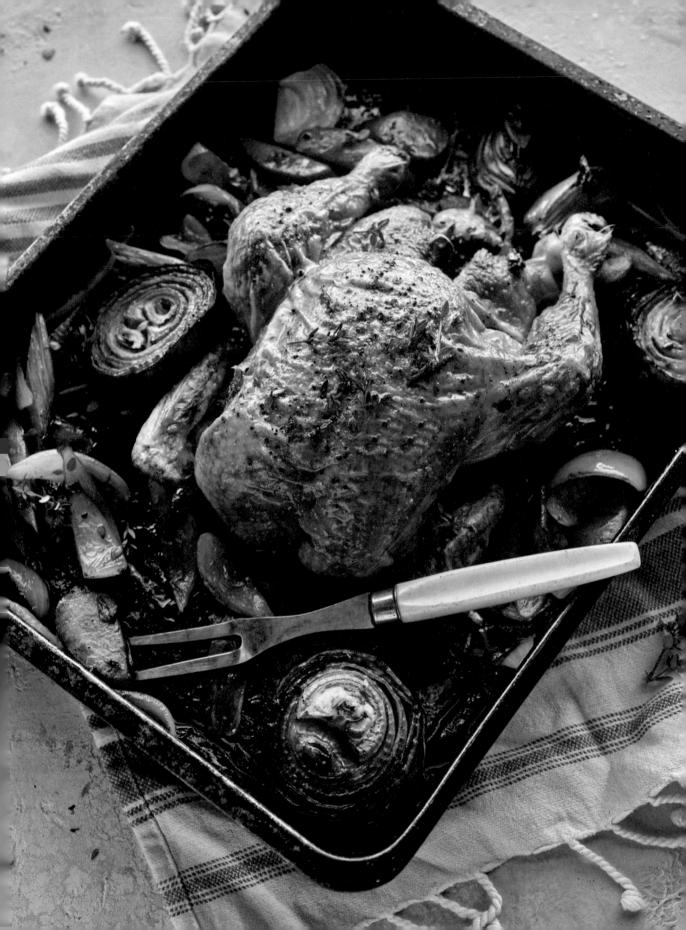

# CREAMY CHICKEN AND MUSHROOM RAGOUT

This is very reasonable in calories and yet it feels very indulgent at the same time. If you would like to bulk up the meal and the nutrition, serve it with a big bowl of blanched broccoli and peas. A true hug for your belly!

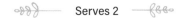 Serves 2

low-calorie cooking spray

salt and black pepper

2 boneless, skinless
    chicken breasts

1 white onion, diced

100g button mushrooms,
    sliced

1 garlic clove, crushed

1 chicken stock cube

250ml boiling water

100g reduced-fat crème
    fraîche

½ lemon, juiced

1 tsp chopped fresh thyme,
    plus extra to garnish

boiled rice, boiled baby
    potatoes or baked sweet
    potatoes, to serve

Heat a shallow casserole or a deep frying pan and add some low-calorie cooking spray. Season your chicken breasts with salt and pepper, then add to the pan and cook for 7–10 minutes, turning over halfway through, until golden brown on both sides. Add your onion, mushrooms and garlic and fry gently until softened.

Dissolve the stock cube in the hot water, then pour into the pan and simmer for 15 minutes, until the chicken is fully cooked. Remove from the heat and gently stir in your crème fraîche, lemon juice and thyme. Do not put the pan back on the heat now, as this will cause the sauce to split.

Garnish with a few fresh thyme leaves and serve with boiled rice, boiled baby potatoes or baked sweet potatoes.

**Nutritional Information**

|  | Per Serving |
| --- | --- |
| Calories | 370kcal |
| Protein | 36g |
| Carbohydrates | 18g |
| Fat | 16g |

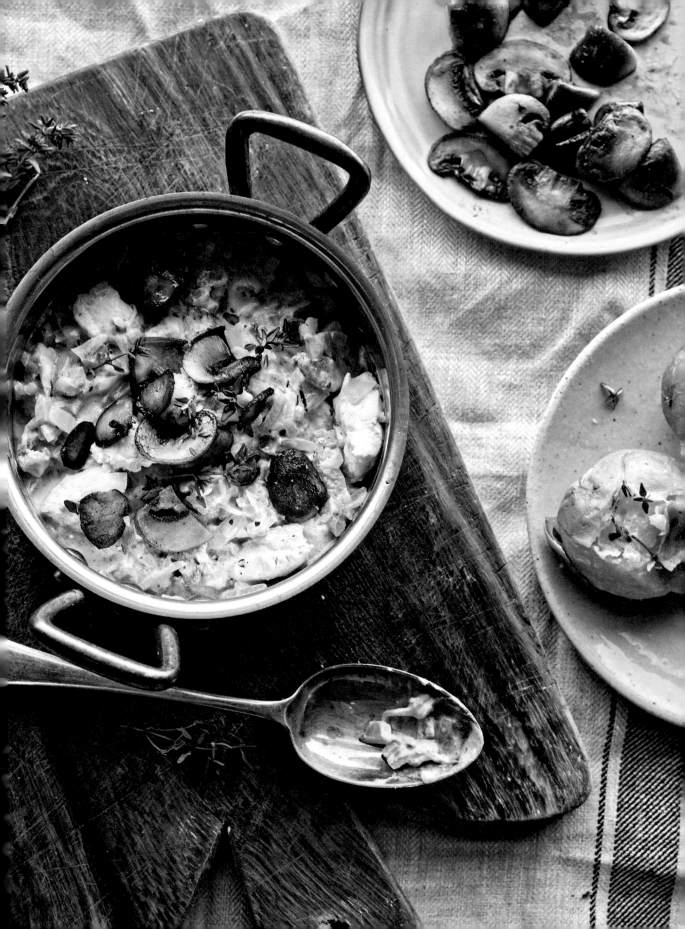

# GARLIC-CRUMBED CHICKEN SCHNITZEL

This is a well-balanced, nutritious dish. The key is to flatten the chicken so that it cooks quicker and more evenly and keeps its juices. I serve this with some guacamole (page 173) or a tomato salsa.

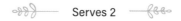 Serves 2

2 chicken breasts,
   butterflied
150g breadcrumbs (panko
   are the best IMO)
1 tbsp garlic powder
olive oil
guacamole (page 173) or
   tomato salsa, to serve

Place a sheet of parchment paper on the counter and place one chicken breast on top. Cover with a second sheet of parchment paper, then using a kitchen hammer or a heavy-based pan, whack the chicken until it becomes flat and even.

Mix your breadcrumbs and garlic powder together in a wide, shallow bowl, then add the chicken, turning to coat.

Put the crumbed chicken back on the parchment paper, cover with the second sheet again and whack again to pound the crumbs into the chicken.

Heat your frying pan and add some olive oil. Add your chicken and fry gently for 3 minutes on each side. Pierce the thickest part of the chicken with the tip of a sharp knife to make sure it's cooked through.

Serve with guacamole or tomato salsa on the side.

### Nutritional Information

|  | Per Serving |
| --- | --- |
| Calories | 554kcal |
| Protein | 49g |
| Carbohydrates | 55g |
| Fat | 15g |

# LUCY'S CRISPY CHICKEN BITES

My wonderful niece Lucy is really into cooking, whereas my other nieces, Amy, Eva and Ellie, are more into it being served up to them! When Lucy started cooking, I was blown away that at just nine years of age she is so good at it. Her timing is wonderful and all her dishes are gorgeous. I asked her to create a simple recipe for me and this is what she did.
It is UNREAL and tastes of more!

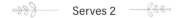 Serves 2

Preheat your oven to 200°C. Line a baking tray with non-stick baking paper.

Put your cornflakes in a blender or a large bowl and blitz or crush into a powder. The more you crush, the finer the powder will be. Stir in your paprika and garlic powder and season well, then tip out into a wide, shallow bowl.

Crack an egg into a second wide, shallow bowl and whisk in your milk.

Pop your chicken strips in the egg mixture and turn to coat well. Remove and shake off any excess egg mixture, then pop into the cornflake mixture and turn to coat evenly.

Place the chicken on a baking tray and cook in the preheated oven for 15 minutes. Remove from the oven and shake them around on the tray, then return to the oven and cook for another 15 minutes. The thinner your strips, the less cooking time they will need, so always check that the chicken is cooked by cutting through the thickest part to make sure there are no traces of pink. Serve hot.

100g cornflakes

1 tsp paprika

1 tsp garlic powder

salt and black pepper

1 egg

2 tsp low-fat milk

2 boneless, skinless
   chicken breasts, sliced
   into strips

**Nutritional Information**

| | Per Serving |
| --- | --- |
| Calories | 364kcal |
| Protein | 30g |
| Carbohydrates | 44g |
| Fat | 7g |

# THAI GREEN CHICKEN CURRY

This is so delicious but also very healthy. The paste can last for up to four weeks in the fridge as long as you keep it in an airtight jar. The more paste you add to your curry, the spicier it will be. I always add mine at the last minute so it will hold onto its bright, vibrant colour. I cook my chicken from raw in the coconut milk, as it provides a much more tender end product.

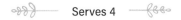 Serves 4

400g boneless, skinless chicken, sliced into strips

1 x 400ml tin of reduced-fat coconut milk

1 chicken stock cube

100g frozen petit pois

100g mangetout, chopped

100g green beans, chopped

2–3 spring onions, sliced

handful of fresh coriander, chopped
(reserve some for garnish)

1 fresh red chilli, deseeded and finely chopped,
to garnish

1 lime, cut into wedges, to serve

boiled basmati rice, to serve

**For the paste:**

2 shallots, chopped

2 sticks of lemongrass, bashed and chopped

4 garlic cloves, chopped

2.5cm piece of fresh ginger, peeled and chopped

4 fresh green chillies, deseeded and chopped

6 lime leaves

50g fresh basil (stalks and all)

50g fresh coriander (stalks and all)

1 tbsp shrimp paste (I order this online from Mr. Bells)

1 tsp ground cumin

1 tsp ground coriander

2 tsp sesame oil

To make the paste, pop everything into a NutriBullet or high-speed blender and blitz until smooth.

Put your chicken strips, coconut milk and chicken stock cube in a large pan and bring to the boil, then reduce the heat and simmer for 10 minutes, until the chicken is cooked through.

Add your petit pois, mangetout and green beans and simmer for 5 minutes.

Add 4 tsp of your paste, then stir in the spring onions and most of the coriander at the last minute. Garnish with the fresh red chilli and reserved fresh coriander and serve with lime wedges and boiled basmati rice.

**Nutritional Information**

|  | Per Serving |
|---|---|
| Calories | 328kcal |
| Protein | 29g |
| Carbohydrates | 19g |
| Fat | 15g |

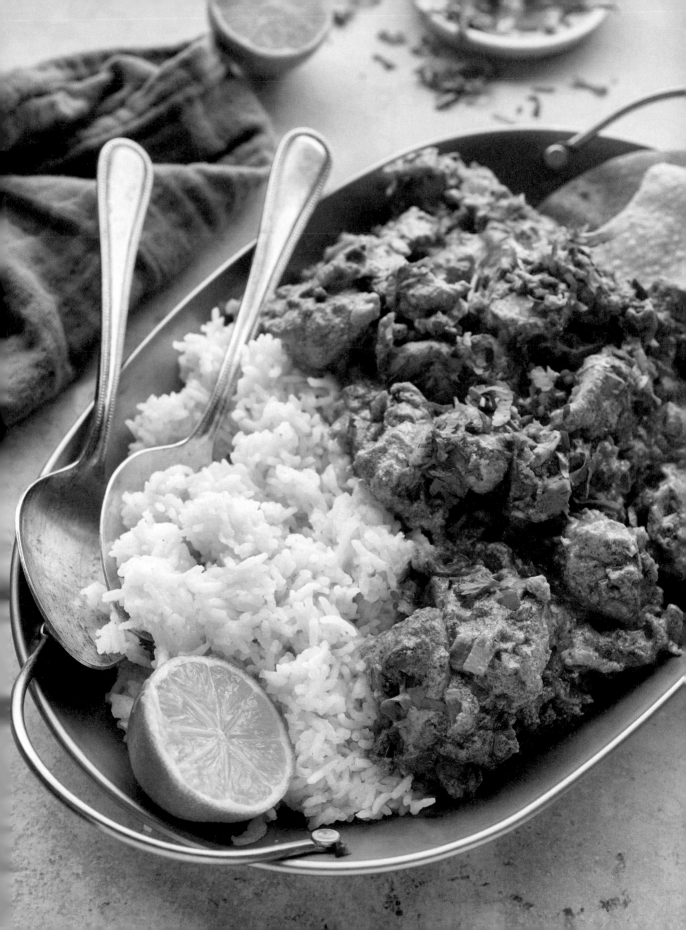

# INDIAN BUTTER CHICKEN

I honestly think that this is just as nice as the real thing, but my version is super healthy. It's high in protein and carbohydrates and low in fat, and ironically this butter chicken doesn't have any butter in it! To really get the flavours going, marinate your chicken the day before.

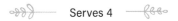 Serves 4

200g low-fat natural yoghurt

1 lemon, juiced

2 tsp ground cumin

2 tsp smoked paprika

2 tsp garam masala

500g boneless, skinless chicken
  breasts, cut into bite-sized
  pieces

olive oil

2 white onions, diced

3 garlic cloves, finely chopped

1 fresh green chilli, deseeded
  and thinly sliced

2 tsp ginger purée or 1 x 2.5cm
  piece of fresh ginger, peeled
  and chopped

1 tbsp tomato purée

2 chicken stock cubes

250ml boiling water

fresh coriander leaves, to
  garnish

boiled basmati rice, to serve

poppadums, to serve

mango chutney, to serve

Put the yoghurt, lemon juice, cumin, smoked paprika and garam masala in a large bowl and stir to combine, then add the chicken and stir again to coat. Cover the bowl with cling film and marinate in the fridge overnight.

The next day, heat a large frying pan and add some oil. Add your onions, garlic, chilli and ginger and sauté for 2 minutes.

Dissolve your stock cubes in the hot water, then pour this into the pan and add the tomato purée. Simmer for 6 minutes.

Add your marinated chicken and simmer for 10 minutes, until the chicken is cooked through.

Garnish with fresh coriander leaves and serve with boiled basmati rice and some poppadums and mango chutney on the side.

**Nutritional Information**

|  | Per Serving |
| --- | --- |
| Calories | 401kcal |
| Protein | 37g |
| Carbohydrates | 50g |
| Fat | 6g |

# CHICKEN MASALA

Using butter in a weight loss book seems a bit mad, doesn't it? But it's all about moderation and not treating food as good or bad. Food is food, and as an Irish person, I think that butter is awesome. We have such amazing pastures here that I couldn't not have real butter in the book. This one is such a lovely dish and served with some fluffy rice you are just going to be in heaven. Like the tikka masala in my last book, this may seem like a long list of ingredients, but once combined, this is simple to make.

Serves 4

Melt your butter in a large pan or heavy-based casserole. Add your onions and garlic and gently sauté until soft.

Add all your spices and cook for 30 seconds, until fragrant. Add your fresh tomatoes and tomato purée and cook for 3 minutes.

Add your milk and chicken and cook gently for 15 minutes, until the chicken is lightly poached. This keeps your chicken lovely and soft.

Stir in your cream, then add your spring onions and chopped coriander and season with salt and pepper. Serve with some fluffy rice and garnish with fresh coriander leaves.

60g butter

2 onions, finely diced

2 garlic cloves, chopped

2 tsp ground ginger

2 tsp garam masala

2 tsp curry powder

1 tsp ground coriander

1 tsp chilli powder

½ tsp ground turmeric

2 ripe tomatoes, chopped small

1 tsp tomato purée

200ml low-fat milk

4 boneless, skinless chicken breasts, cut into strips

60ml light cream

2 spring onions, thinly sliced

2 tsp chopped fresh coriander, plus extra whole leaves to garnish

salt and black pepper

boiled basmati rice, to serve

## Nutritional Information

|  | Per Serving |
| --- | --- |
| Calories | 360kcal |
| Protein | 31g |
| Carbohydrates | 15g |
| Fat | 19g |
| Gluten Free | ✔ |

# LEMON AND GARLIC CHICKEN SKEWERS

Having chicken every day can be boring, but these are so simple and have so much flavour. Plus they're very high in protein, so they're a good snack option if you're looking to increase your protein intake. They're also ideal for a party, as they are easy to eat and not messy.

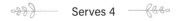 Serves 4

1 lemon, zested and juiced

4 garlic cloves, finely chopped

2 sprigs of fresh rosemary, finely chopped

4 tsp honey

2 tsp olive oil

salt and black pepper

4 boneless, skinless chicken breasts

Mix your lemon zest and juice, garlic, rosemary, honey, olive oil and some salt and pepper in a large bowl.

Cut each chicken breast into three large chunks, then add to the bowl and stir to coat in the marinade. Cover the bowl with cling film and marinate in the fridge for at least 4 hours or overnight.

Meanwhile, soak 12 wooden skewers in cold water for 2 hours – this will prevent them from burning and chipping. Or you can use metal skewers if you have them.

Preheat your oven to 200°C.

Skewer each piece of chicken and place on a baking tray. Cook in the preheated oven for 10 minutes, then turn each skewer over and cook for another 15 minutes. Serve hot.

**Nutritional Information**

|  | Per Serving |
| --- | --- |
| Calories | 176kcal |
| Protein | 23g |
| Carbohydrates | 29g |
| Fat | 5g |
| Gluten Free | ✔ |

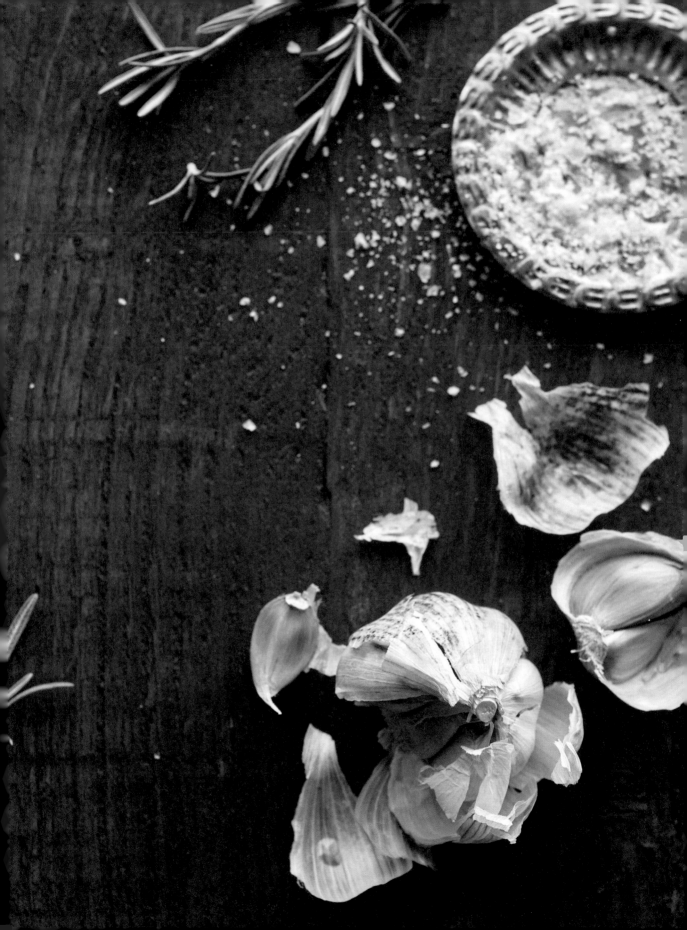

# ROAST LAMB
## WITH MINT AND GARLIC CRUST

A classic Sunday lunch with no fuss and the simplest accompaniment that will highlight the flavour of the meat. A leg of lamb will be the most flavoursome cut of meat but can be a little tricky to carve, so I usually go for a boned and rolled leg of lamb. If you're getting this from a butcher, ask them to trim the fat off to reduce the calories even more. Sometimes I like to add some sweet potatoes cut into thick slices to the roasting tray too.

Serves 6

1 x 1.6kg boned and rolled leg of lamb
2 onions, halved or cut into wedges
2 garlic cloves, peeled and left whole
2 sweet potatoes, sliced into discs
sprig of fresh rosemary
sprig of fresh thyme
salt and black pepper
100ml water

**For the mint and garlic crust:**
1 shallot, halved lengthways
4 garlic cloves, peeled
30g fresh mint (including the stalks –
   they're full of flavour!)
1 tbsp Dijon mustard
1 tbsp lemon juice
2 tsp olive oil

Preheat your oven to 180°C.

Half an hour before you're ready to start cooking, take your lamb out of the fridge to bring it up to room temperature.

To make the crust, place all the ingredients in a food processor or blender and blitz into a rough, chunky paste. Set aside.

Scatter your chunky chopped vegetables, rosemary and thyme and whole garlic cloves in a roasting tray (this is the trivet) and pop your lamb on top. Spread the mint and garlic crust on top of the lamb and season well with salt and pepper. Pour your water around the vegetables.

Cook in the preheated oven for 1 hour for medium rare, 1 hour 20 minutes for medium and 1 hour 40 minutes for well done. Leave to rest for 10 minutes before carving and serving.

**Nutritional Information**

|  | Per Serving |
| --- | --- |
| Calories | 775kcal |
| Protein | 80g |
| Carbohydrates | 24g |
| Fat | 39g |
| Gluten Free | ✔ |

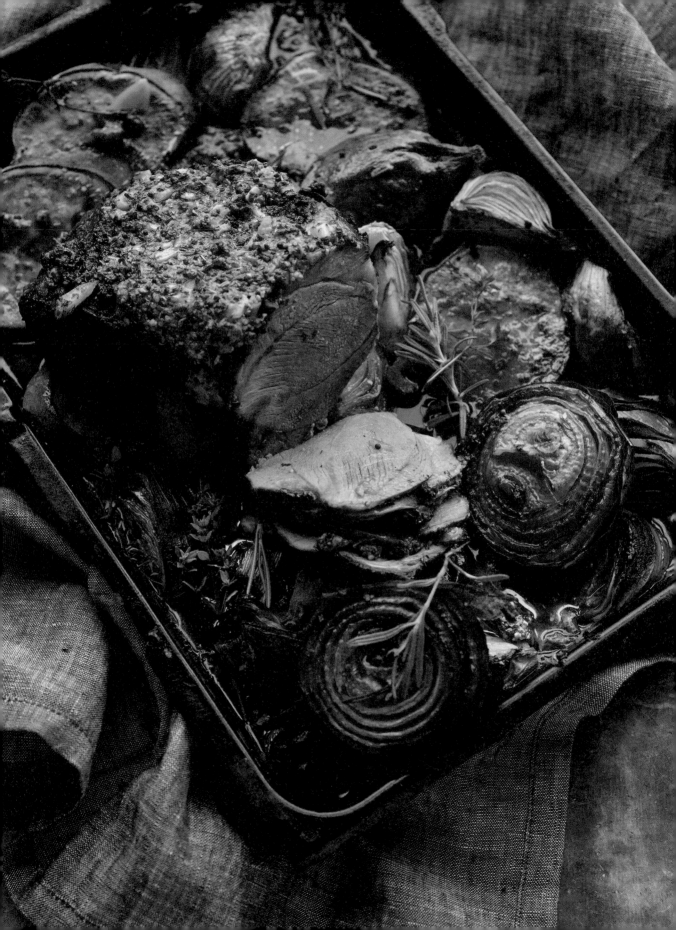

# CRISPY TUNA CAKES

This is a handy recipe for those times when you think you have nothing to eat. This is made with staples that we all have in the fridge and is a cool twist on a toasted tuna special! I serve this with some rocket salad, but if you would like to make it into a more substantial meal, add some of the spicy wedges from page 181. I use tinned tuna as it holds its structure in the mixture better.

### Serves 4

400g Maris Piper potatoes, peeled and cut into cubes

200g tinned tuna, drained

1 white onion, finely chopped

60g reduced-fat crème fraîche

40g light red Cheddar cheese, grated

10g fresh chives, chopped

salt and black pepper

30g plain flour

1 large egg

1 tsp low-fat milk

40g breadcrumbs

20g butter

olive oil

lighter-than-light mayonnaise, to serve

squeeze of lemon, to serve

Put the potatoes in a pan of cold water and bring to the boil, then reduce the heat and cook for 12 minutes, until completely cooked through. Drain and mash well, getting as many lumps out to make it as smooth as possible.

Pop the mashed potatoes into a large bowl and add your tuna, onion, crème fraîche, grated cheese and chives. Season with salt and pepper and mix well to combine.

Divide into eight mounds and flatten each one down. Shape with the edge of your knife into a neat square. Set up three wide, shallow bowls. Put the flour in one bowl. Put the egg and milk in the second bowl and whisk together. Put the breadcrumbs in the last bowl.

Using one hand (so that you keep your other hand dry), place one of your squares first into the flour, then the egg, then the breadcrumbs.

Heat a non-stick frying pan and add the butter and a little olive oil. Working in batches, add some squares to the pan and fry for 3 minutes on each side, until golden brown and heated through.

Mix a squeeze of lemon juice with some mayonnaise and serve alongside the tuna melts.

## Nutritional Information

|  | Per Serving |
| --- | --- |
| Calories | 388kcal |
| Protein | 24g |
| Carbohydrates | 30g |
| Fat | 19g |

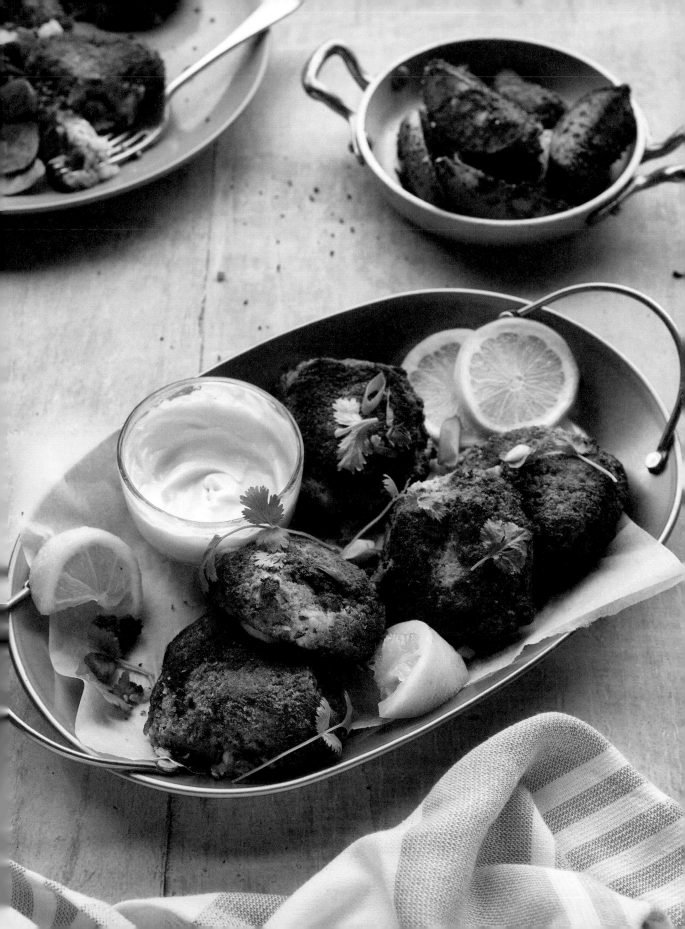

# THAI-STYLE FISH CAKES

Pan-fried fish cakes can be messy, which is why I favour this style more. They are moist and just bursting with flavour. I love serving mine with my spicy potato wedges (page 181) and a little lighter-than-light mayo. Don't be afraid to try these, as they're so easy to make and such a crowd pleaser! The egg gives the cakes a light, mousse-like texture.

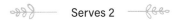 Serves 2

300g fresh salmon, skinned, boned
  and chopped into chunks
1 medium free-range egg
1 stick of lemongrass, bashed and
  chopped finely
1 fresh red chilli, deseeded and chopped
1 tbsp Thai red curry paste
1 tsp fish sauce
salt and black pepper
50g green beans, finely chopped
  (I use frozen for convenience)
low-calorie cooking spray
fresh coriander leaves, to garnish
1 lemon, cut into wedges, to serve
lighter-than-light mayonnaise, to serve
spicy potato wedges (page 181), to serve

Pop your salmon, egg, lemongrass, chilli, curry paste, fish sauce and some salt and pepper in a NutriBullet or food processor and blitz into a paste.

Transfer into a bowl and mix in your finely chopped green beans. Refrigerate for up to one day, until ready to use.

When it's time to cook, simply divide the mixture into portions and shape into cakes. Heat your frying pan and add some low-calorie cooking spray. Add two or three fish cakes (depending on how large your pan is – you might need to cook them in batches) and cook for 3 minutes on one side, until golden brown. Flip over and continue to fry until the fish cakes are cooked through and golden brown on the second side too.

Garnish with fresh coriander leaves and serve with lemon wedges, mayo and spicy potato wedges on the side.

### Nutritional Information

|  | Per Serving |
| --- | --- |
| Calories | 422kcal |
| Protein | 37g |
| Carbohydrates | 11g |
| Fat | 24g |
| Gluten Free | ✔ |

# POACHED SALMON

This is my favourite way to have salmon, as it's just so subtle and delicate. I also love it because you can have it the next day or have it cooked ahead of time for a nice salmon platter if you're having guests over or a communion party, etc. Poaching is a method in which you cook the salmon in lightly simmering water that has some flavouring in it. Simples! I would serve this with some lovely boiled potatoes and the salsa verde from page 177.

Serves 4

Fill a deep pan with cold water and add your lemon slices, bay leaves and peppercorns. Bring to a gentle simmer.

Pop in your salmon and cover with a lid. Gently poach for 8 minutes, until the salmon is cooked through. Serve hot or cold.

2 lemons, sliced

2 bay leaves

4 black peppercorns

4 x 200g salmon fillets, boned (ask your fishmonger to do this for you)

### Nutritional Information

| | Per Serving |
|---|---|
| Calories | 300kcal |
| Protein | 48g |
| Carbohydrates | 2g |
| Fat | 11g |
| Gluten Free | ✔ |

# 'STEAMED' ASIAN-STYLE SALMON

In the past, whenever I came across a recipe that called for a steamer I wouldn't make it because I don't have one at home, so let me show you this method. It doesn't require a steamer but it creates the same effect. The water in the tin foil parcel creates the steam and cooks the fish without adding any extra oil. Remove the skin from the salmon to shave off another few calories. You can also use the paste with beef, chicken or prawns. I love this salmon because you can have it with rice and veg for dinner and the next day you can have it cold for a salad, so it's amazing for batch cooking.

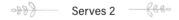 Serves 2

1 bunch of fresh coriander
   (stalks and all)
10 fresh mint leaves
3 garlic cloves, peeled
1 fresh red chilli, deseeded and
   diced
2 limes, juiced, plus extra
   wedges to serve
1 tbsp sesame oil
1 tsp sea salt
1 tsp fish sauce
2 x 180g salmon fillets, skinned
   and boned
splash of water
fresh coriander and shredded
   carrot salad, to serve

Preheat your oven to 200°C.

Put all your ingredients except for the water and salmon in a food processor, NutriBullet or high-speed blender and blitz into a fine paste.

Place two large sheets of tin foil on your counter, then put a salmon fillet in the middle of each one. Spread the salmon with the paste and start creating a parcel shape with the tin foil. Add about 2 teaspoons of water to each parcel and close tightly so that no steam can escape while the salmon cooks.

Pop the parcels onto a baking tray, then cook in the preheated oven for 12–15 minutes, until cooked through. You know salmon is cooked when it flakes apart easily when you gently press it.

This salmon can be served hot or cold. I like to have it with lime wedges and a simple salad of fresh coriander and shredded carrot and any extra herb paste on the side.

## Nutritional Information

|  | Per Serving |
| --- | --- |
| Calories | 602kcal |
| Protein | 41g |
| Carbohydrates | 15g |
| Fat | 42g |
| Gluten Free | ✔ |

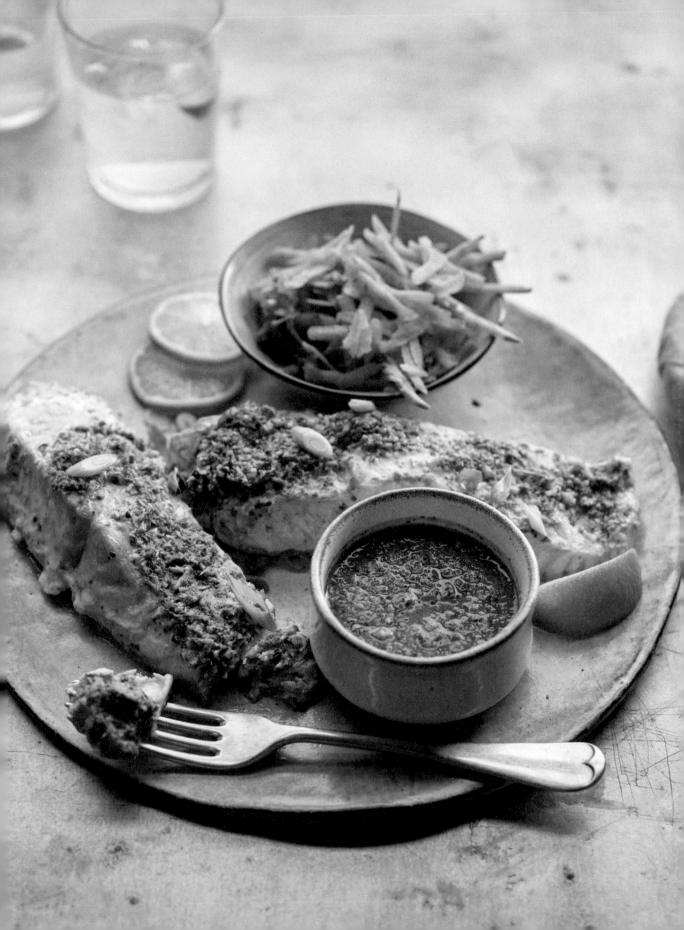

# SICILIAN FISH STEW

Sometimes we don't eat fish because it can be bland and boring, but this stew is so tasty and simple to make. You can use cod, pollock or monkfish in this dish, but I always prefer to use hake rather than cod, as I find it to be so much more flavoursome.
A good firm white fish is what is needed.

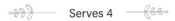 Serves 4

4 x 200g hake fillets
  (or any firm white fish)
salt and black pepper
low-calorie cooking spray
1 red onion, sliced
2 red peppers, diced
2 green peppers, diced
3 garlic cloves, crushed
25ml balsamic vinegar
1 tsp brown sugar
1 x 500g carton of passata
1 x 400g tin of chopped tomatoes
4 tbsp tomato purée
2 tbsp capers, drained
1 lemon, cut into wedges, to garnish
boiled basmati rice or sweet potato
  wedges, to serve

Pat your hake dry with kitchen paper, then season with salt and pepper.

Heat a non-stick frying pan and add some low-calorie cooking spray. Add the hake to the pan, skin side down, and cook for 2 minutes, until golden brown. Remove from the pan and set aside.

Heat a large saucepan and add some low-calorie cooking spray. Add your onion, red and green peppers, garlic, balsamic vinegar and sugar. This is called a gastrique and it provides a contrast of sweet and sour flavour to the base of your dish. Gently sauté until the onion and peppers are softened.

Add your passata, chopped tomatoes, tomato purée and capers and bring to the boil. Reduce the heat and simmer for 5 minutes.

Pop your fish on top with the skin facing up and simmer for 15 minutes, until the fish is cooked through.

Ladle into warmed bowls and garnish with lemon wedges. Serve with rice or roasted sweet potato wedges.

## Nutritional Information

| | Per Serving |
|---|---|
| Calories | 280kcal |
| Protein | 41g |
| Carbohydrates | 22g |
| Fat | 3g |
| Gluten Free | ✔ |

# GREEK-STYLE ROASTED COD
## WITH PAPRIKA, OLIVES, LEMON AND GARLIC

This is a beautiful dish that's so simple. I love the skin on fish and I never remove it,
but I understand if you don't like it, so if you would like to remove it, work away.
It won't affect the end dish. Cod is a white, meaty, flaky fish with a mild flavour,
so it adapts well to strong ingredients.

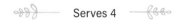 Serves 4

Preheat your oven to 200°C.

Mix together your flour, lemon zest, paprika, cumin,
coriander and some salt and pepper in a bowl. Set aside.

Heat a deep ovenproof frying pan and add your olive oil,
lemon juice, garlic and butter. Bring to a simmer for 5
minutes, then add your fish and green olives.

Dust the spiced flour on top of each piece of fish, then
add the fish to the pan along with your rosemary.

Transfer the pan to the preheated oven and cook for
10–12 minutes. Pierce a knife into the middle of a piece of
cod and check that it's hot, as this will indicate it's fully
cooked through.

To serve, pop the fish on top of a bed of rice and garnish
with lemon wedges and a sprig of rosemary, then pour
the juices from the pan over the top.

40g plain flour

1 lemon, zested

1 tsp smoked paprika

1 tsp ground cumin

1 tsp ground coriander

salt and black pepper

80ml olive oil

80ml lemon juice

5 garlic cloves, chopped

15g butter

4 x 200g cod fillets, skinned
and boned

10 green olives, pitted and
sliced

2 sprigs of fresh rosemary, plus
extra for garnish

1 lemon, cut into wedges, for
garnish

boiled basmati rice, to serve

### Nutritional Information

|  | Per Serving |
| --- | --- |
| Calories | 413kcal |
| Protein | 27g |
| Carbohydrates | 13g |
| Fat | 28g |

# PAN-FRIED HAKE
## WITH BUTTER BEANS, BACON AND SPINACH

If I had to choose between cod and hake, I would always pick hake. No disrespect to cod, but I find that hake has a lot more flavour and a nicer texture. This is a really simple, healthy, nutritious one-pot wonder that's full of protein. People are often afraid to cook fish, but it's so easy. I always seal it on a pan and either finish it in the oven or under the grill, as that way you have more control in the cooking.

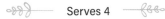 Serves 4

4 tsp olive oil, plus extra for cooking

4 x 180g hake fillets, skin on and deboned

salt and black pepper

150g smoked bacon lardons

1 red onion, diced

2 garlic cloves, diced

1 fresh red chilli, deseeded and diced

2 tsp smoked paprika

2 x 400g tins of butter beans, drained and rinsed

400g spinach (don't worry, it will wilt down!)

2 lemons

1 fresh red chilli, deseeded and thinly sliced, to garnish

fresh chives, to garnish

Preheat your grill.

Heat an ovenproof non-stick frying pan and add a splash of olive oil. Season your hake fillets with salt and pepper, then add to the pan, skin side down. Cook for 1 minute to seal the skin, then place the pan under the grill and cook for 7 minutes, until the fish is cooked from the top all the way down to the bottom. Flip over, then set aside and keep warm.

Heat a separate large frying pan and add the bacon lardons (you don't need to add any oil). Fry until the fat has rendered out of the bacon, then add your onion, garlic, chilli and paprika and sauté for 4 minutes, until the bacon crisps.

Add your 4 teaspoons of olive oil and the butter beans and cook for 2 minutes. Juice one of the lemons, then add the juice to the pan along with the spinach. Pop a lid on top so your spinach wilts faster. Season with salt and pepper.

To serve, cut the remaining lemon into wedges. Put the hake on a bed of butter beans and garnish with lemon wedges, red chilli and chives.

### Nutritional Information

|  | Per Serving |
| --- | --- |
| Calories | 516kcal |
| Protein | 53g |
| Carbohydrates | 26g |
| Fat | 22g |
| Gluten Free | ✔ |

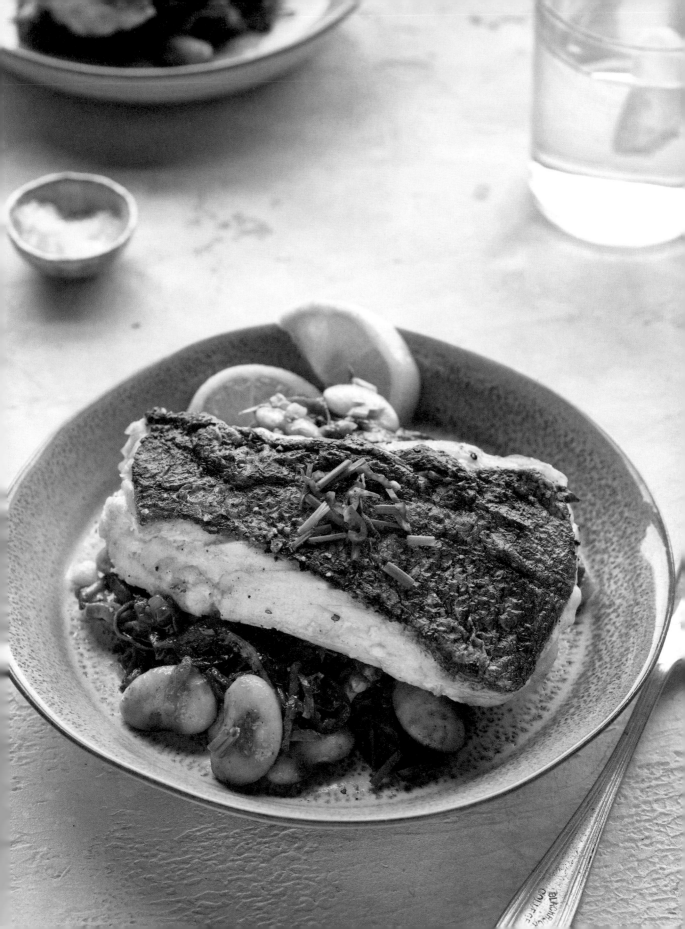

# LIME AND COCONUT TIGER PRAWNS

As I sit here writing this book in the middle of a pandemic, I'm dreaming of eating prawns pil pil on a beach in Spain with the sun beating down on me. I've given this classic Mediterranean dish a tropical twist by adding lime and coconut for a zesty, nutty flavour that adds extra oomph. Don't add the herbs until the very end, as overcooking them will cause them to blacken and go sour and you don't want that!

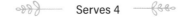 Serves 4

1 tbsp extra virgin olive oil

4 garlic cloves, crushed

1 fresh red chilli, deseeded and finely diced

20 large tiger prawns

4 spring onions, thinly sliced

20g desiccated coconut or flakes

1 lime, juiced

1 tbsp chopped fresh coriander, plus extra to garnish

1 lemon, cut into wedges, to serve

1 fresh red chilli, deseeded and finely chopped, to garnish

warm ciabatta bread, to serve

Heat a large frying pan and add just a drop of olive oil. Add the garlic and start to lightly fry. Once the garlic starts to turn golden, add the remaining tablespoon of oil and reduce the heat. Pop in your chilli and prawns and cook gently just until the prawns change colour and turn light pink.

Add your spring onions, coconut, lime juice and coriander, and stir through.

Serve immediately with lemon wedges to squeeze over for extra zing and garnish with the fresh red chilli and extra coriander. Mop up the pan with the warm ciabatta bread to get all those bits eaten!

## Nutritional Information

|  | Per Serving |
| --- | --- |
| Calories | 245kcal |
| Protein | 17g |
| Carbohydrates | 12g |
| Fat | 14g |

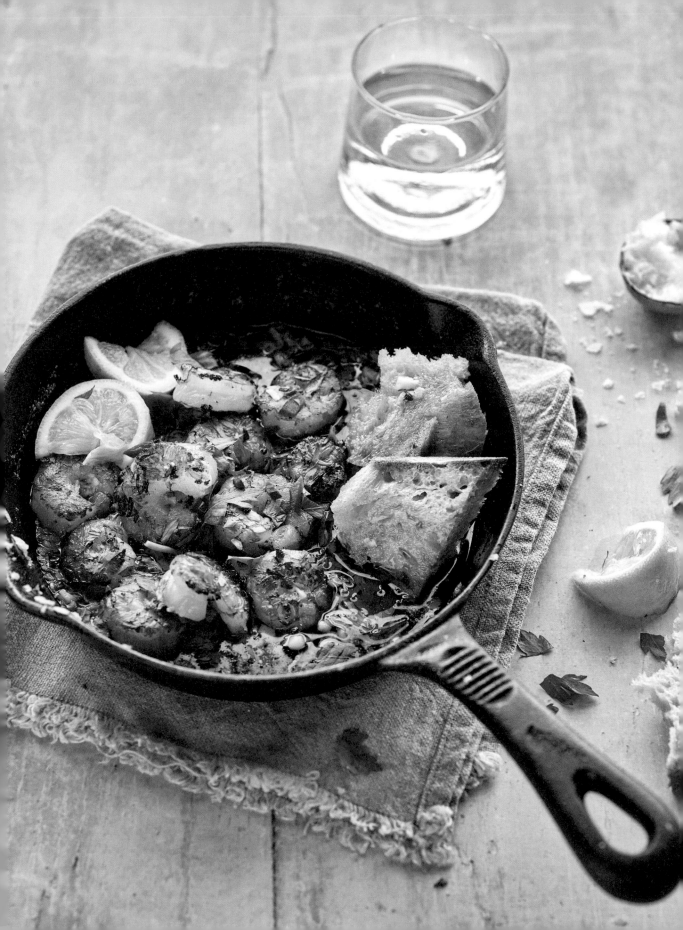

# HOMEMADE MUSHROOM, GARLIC AND MOZZARELLA PIZZA

Now when I say that this is delicious, I'm not joking! The mushrooms should be nice and cooked before you pop them on the pizza. The earthiness of the mushrooms, softness of the mozzarella and sharpness of the passata is a match made in heaven! When you are pan frying the pizza, try to char the base a little bit!

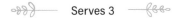 Serves 3

100g plain flour, plus extra for dusting

100g 0% fat natural yoghurt

cracked black pepper

olive oil

10 button mushrooms, sliced

2 spring onions, thinly sliced

2 garlic cloves, chopped

50g passata

125g light mozzarella, thinly sliced

rocket, to garnish

chilli flakes, to garnish

Preheat your oven to 180°C.

Put your flour and yoghurt in a bowl and add lots of cracked black pepper. Mix into a dough, then tip out onto a floured surface and divide into three rounds. Using a rolling pin, roll out each base until it's the size of a dinner plate (or the same size as the base of the frying pan you're going to use).

Heat a large frying pan and add some olive oil. Working with one base at a time, fry until golden brown, then flip over and cook until the second side is also golden brown. Set aside.

Meanwhile, heat a separate frying pan and add a little olive oil. Add your mushrooms, spring onions and garlic and sauté until softened.

Spread each of the bases with passata, then top with your mushrooms and the mozzarella. Pop in the oven for 7 minutes, until the cheese has melted.

To serve, garnish with rocket leaves and chilli flakes and cut into slices.

## Nutritional Information

|  | Per Serving |
| --- | --- |
| Calories | 285kcal |
| Protein | 19g |
| Carbohydrates | 32g |
| Fat | 8g |
| Vegetarian | ✔ |

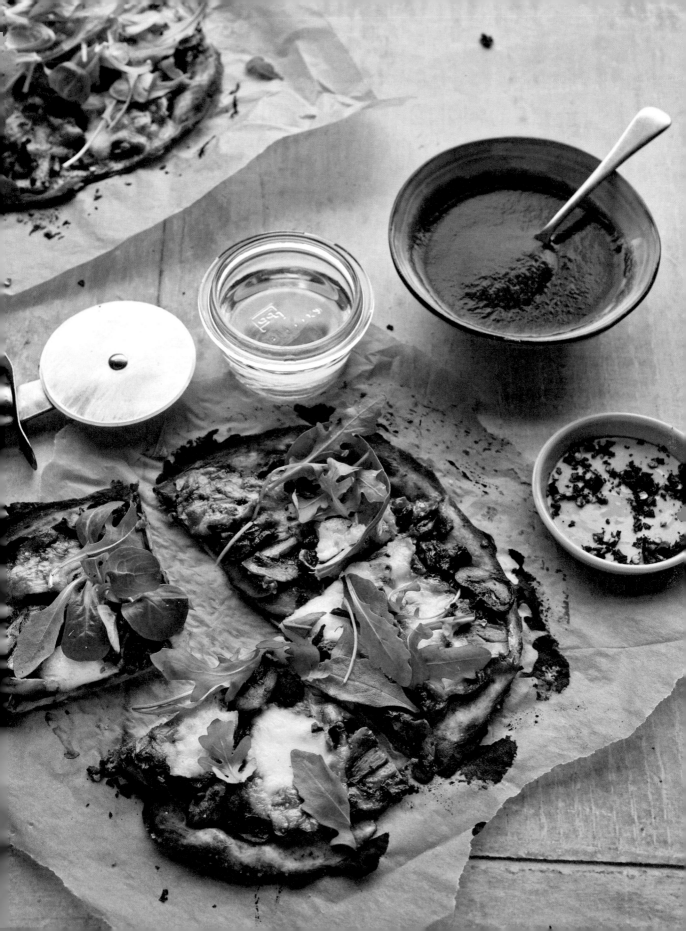

# MEXICAN MIGAS

This is like scrambled eggs on toast, but with a Mexican twist. It's so delicious and packed with flavour. Try serving it with some wholewheat tortillas that you've toasted in a hot oven and cut into strips.

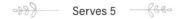 Serves 5

5 tortillas or wraps

1 tbsp olive oil

20g butter

8 eggs, beaten

150g light Cheddar cheese, grated

60g reduced-fat sour cream or
crème fraîche

**FOR THE SALSA:**

1 x 400g tin of black beans,
drained and rinsed

1 red onion, finely chopped

10 cherry tomatoes, quartered

30g fresh coriander, chopped

1 lime, zested and juiced

salt and black pepper

Preheat your oven to 180°C.

Cut your tortillas or wraps into strips and place on a baking tray. Drizzle your olive oil over the strips and toss to coat, then pop them into the preheated oven and bake for 8 minutes, until crisp and golden. Set aside.

To make the salsa, put the black beans, red onion, cherry tomatoes, coriander, lime zest and juice and some salt and pepper in a bowl and stir to combine. Leave out at room temperature to enhance the flavours.

Heat a non-stick frying pan and melt the butter. Stir in your beaten eggs and cook gently until scrambled. Season well.

To assemble, divide the tortilla strips between warmed plates and top with the scrambled eggs, salsa, grated cheese and a spoonful of sour cream or crème fraîche.

### Nutritional Information

|  | Per Serving |
| --- | --- |
| Calories | 585kcal |
| Protein | 27g |
| Carbohydrates | 47g |
| Fat | 31g |
| Vegetarian | ✔ |

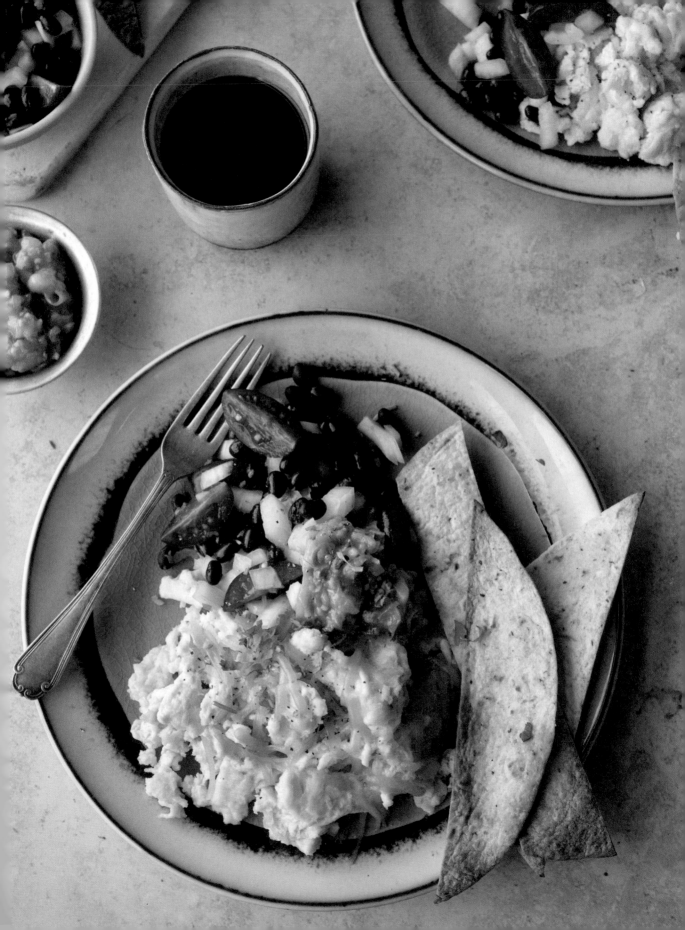

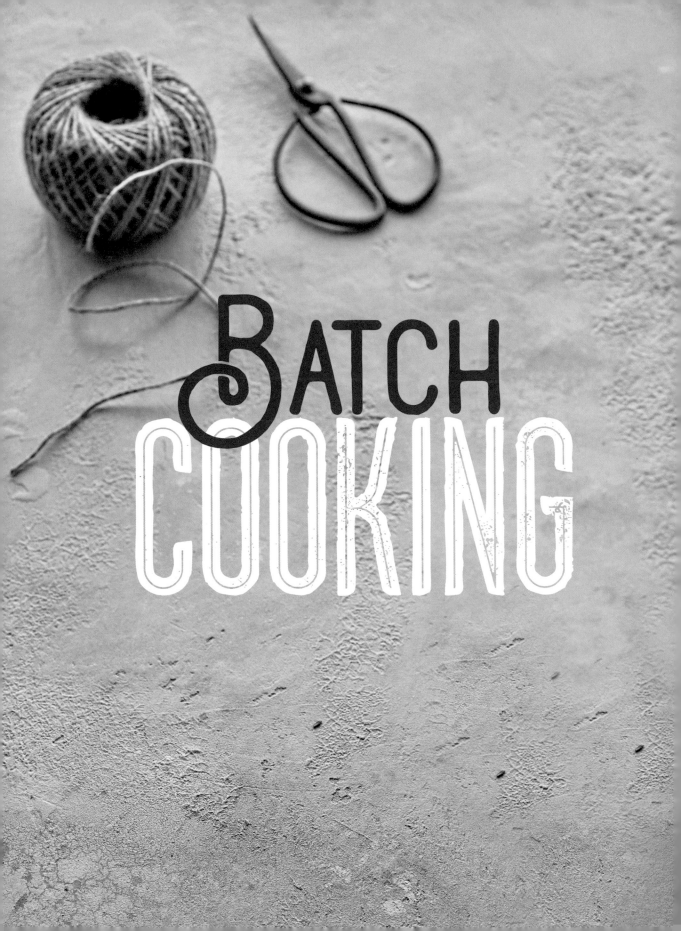

# BATCH COOKING

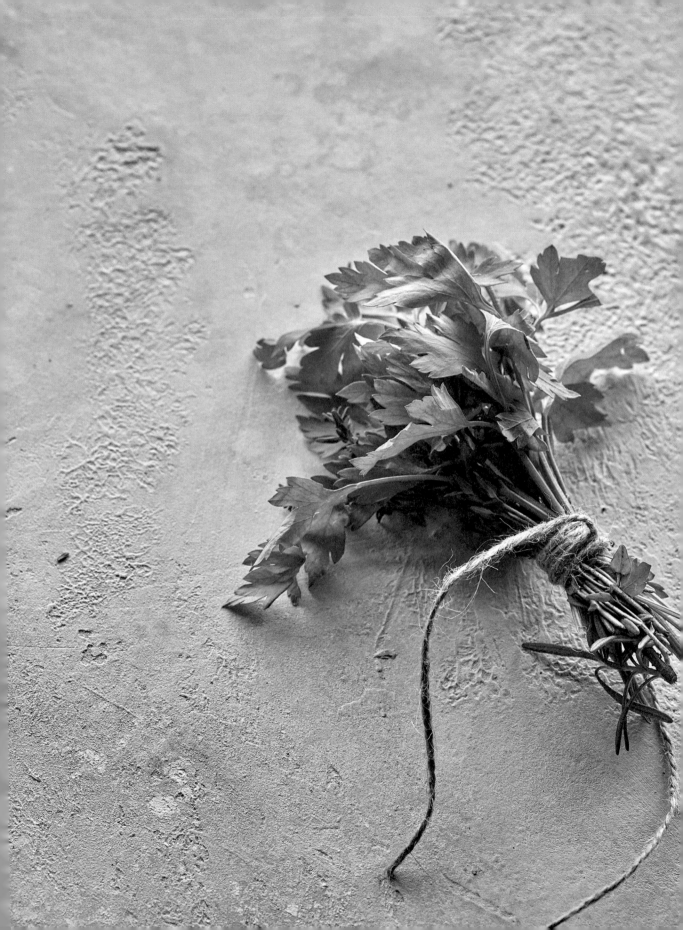

# CHILLI CON CARNE

This is a family favourite, perfect for the smallies and adults too and packed with protein. It's nice to add a few slices of ripe avocado on top, and some sour cream, though that will increase the fat content. This is great for batch cooking as it uses up lots of store cupboard ingredients and keeps for three days in the fridge.

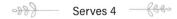 Serves 4

olive oil

1 onion, chopped

1 red pepper, chopped

2 garlic cloves, chopped

450g beef mince (4% fat or less)

1 tsp chilli powder

1 tsp paprika

1 tsp ground cumin

1 x 400g tin of kidney beans, drained and rinsed

½ x 400g tin of chopped tomatoes

30g tomato purée

35g dark chocolate

salt and black pepper

1–2 spring onions, thinly sliced, to garnish

fresh coriander leaves, to garnish

1 lime, cut into wedges, to serve

boiled basmati rice or boiled baby potatoes, to serve

Heat a large saucepan and add some olive oil. Add your onion, red pepper and garlic and lightly sauté until softened.

Add your beef mince and cook until browned all over, breaking up any lumps. Add your chilli powder, paprika and ground cumin and cook for 1 minute, until fragrant.

Add your kidney beans, chopped tomatoes and tomato purée and simmer for 10 minutes, then add your dark chocolate, season with salt and pepper and simmer for 3 minutes.

To serve, ladle into warm bowls and garnish with your spring onions and coriander leaves. Serve the lime wedges on the side. I like to have this with basmati rice, but you can also have it with boiled baby potatoes.

**Nutritional Information**

|  | Per Serving |
| --- | --- |
| Calories | 336kcal |
| Protein | 33g |
| Carbohydrates | 24g |
| Fat | 12g |
| Gluten Free | ✔ |

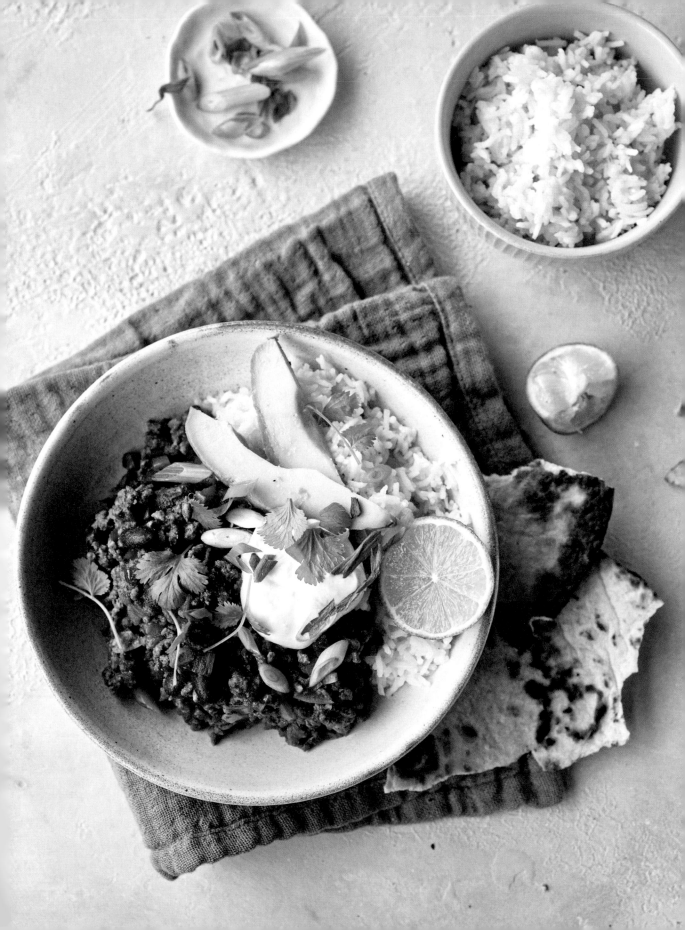

# BAKED AUBERGINE MOUSSAKA

This is a dish that even meat lovers will enjoy! Moussaka is a Greek recipe that's bursting with flavour. I love to have this with a simple dressed salad with fresh cherry tomatoes and crisp raw fennel.

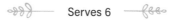 Serves 6

1kg aubergines, thinly sliced into rounds with the skin on

salt and black pepper

60ml olive oil, plus extra for cooking

1 red onion, diced

2 garlic cloves, chopped

2 x 400g tins of chopped tomatoes

1 tbsp tomato purée

50ml water

1 tsp caster sugar

1 tsp cayenne pepper

1 tsp chilli flakes

1 vegetable stock cube

400g light mozzarella cheese, grated

100g light Cheddar cheese, grated

fresh basil leaves, to garnish

## Nutritional Information

|  | Per Serving |
|---|---|
| Calories | 355kcal |
| Protein | 24g |
| Carbohydrates | 18g |
| Fat | 20g |
| Vegetarian | ✔ |

Like the method for the potatoes in the hash browns recipe on page 86, you're going to draw the excess water from the aubergines by salting them. This time, you need to layer the slices in a shallow dish and sprinkle all over with salt. Pop some kitchen paper on top of the aubergines, then put a heavy-based pot on top to help get the excess water out. This should take about 40 minutes.

Meanwhile, to make the marinara sauce, heat a large saucepan and add some olive oil. Add your red onion and garlic and gently sauté until softened.

Stir in the chopped tomatoes, tomato purée, water, sugar, cayenne, chilli flakes and the vegetable stock cube. Simmer for 30 minutes.

Preheat your oven to 190°C.

Heat a large frying pan. Using a pastry brush, lightly brush the aubergine slices with the 60ml of olive oil. Working in batches, gently fry for about 30 seconds on each side to take the edge off the raw texture. Transfer to a plate lined with kitchen paper to remove the excess oil.

In a regular baking dish (a lasagne-type dish is too deep for this recipe), start assembling the moussaka by placing a layer of aubergine slices in the bottom of the dish, then spreading over a layer of sauce and sprinkling on a layer of mozzarella cheese. Repeat the layers until all the ingredients have been used up, then finish with a layer of Cheddar cheese on top.

Bake in the preheated oven for 10 minutes, until the cheese is melted and bubbling on top. Garnish with a few fresh basil leaves and cut into squares to serve.

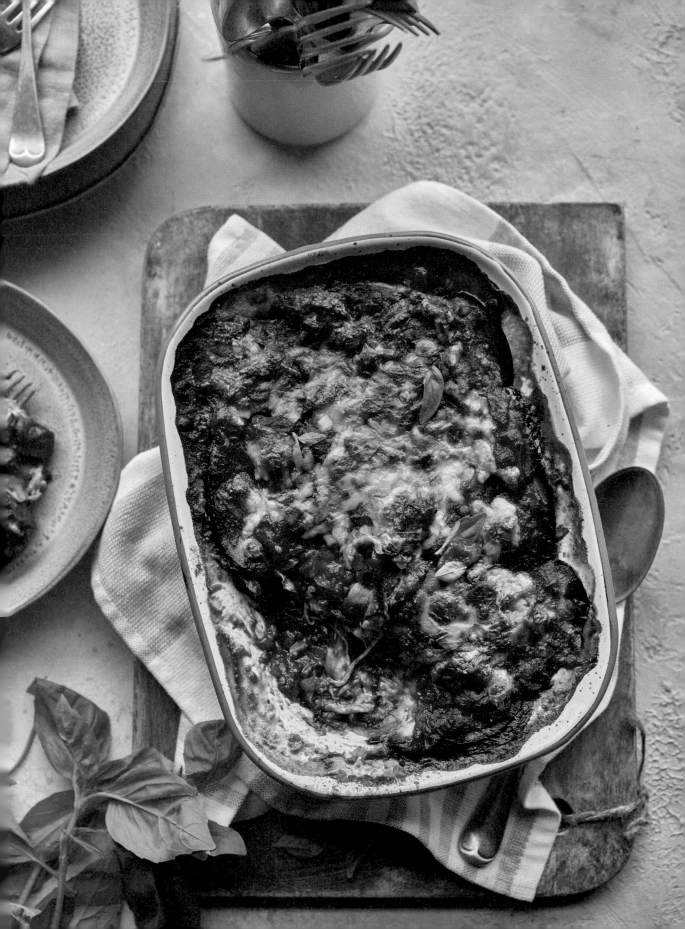

# BEEF STROGANOFF

This is a traditional Russian dish of sautéed beef smothered in a mushroom sauce – basically, stroganoff is a sour cream gravy and I add some paprika for a small change. Make sure you use a prime cut of beef here, as this is the key to a good stroganoff.

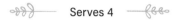 Serves 4

2 tbsp olive oil

500g lean fillet steak, thinly sliced

salt and black pepper

2 onions, diced

15 button mushrooms, sliced

2 garlic cloves, crushed

2 tsp paprika

1 tbsp plain flour

1 tbsp butter

2 beef stock cubes

100ml boiling water

160g reduced-fat crème fraîche

50ml light cream

2 tsp ready-made English mustard

handful of fresh parsley, chopped, plus extra to garnish

boiled baby potatoes or boiled basmati rice, to serve

Heat a large saucepan and add some olive oil. Season your beef strips with salt and pepper, then add to the pan to shallow fry for a few minutes on each side, just until nicely seared. Don't move the pan or stir the beef too much, as this will cause the beef to boil instead of sear.

Add your onions, mushrooms, garlic and paprika and cook for 4 minutes. Stir in your flour and butter and cook for a few minutes – this is a roux, which will thicken the sauce. Dissolve your stock cubes in the hot water, then pour into the pan and simmer for 10 minutes.

Stir in your crème fraîche, cream and mustard and simmer for 5 minutes, then stir in a handful of chopped fresh parsley right at the end.

Serve with boiled baby potatoes or boiled basmati rice and garnish with a little extra parsley.

**Nutritional Information**

|  | Per Serving |
| --- | --- |
| Calories | 410kcal |
| Protein | 31g |
| Carbohydrates | 10g |
| Fat | 27g |

# SHEPHERD'S PIE

For years I didn't realise that the difference between cottage pie and shepherd's pie is that cottage pie uses beef mince and shepherd's pie uses lamb mince. This a great dish because you can batch cook and freeze portions or it will last in the fridge for up to three days. Plus it's packed full of nutrients and covers all your macro and micronutrient needs.

Serves 6

Heat a large saucepan and add some olive oil. Add your onions, carrots, celery and garlic and cook until softened. Add your mince and cook until browned all over, breaking up any lumps. Stir in your flour, Worcestershire sauce, tomato purée and mustard. Dissolve your stock cubes in the hot water, then stir into your lamb mixture and season with salt and pepper. Simmer gently for 1 hour.

Meanwhile, put your potatoes in a pot and cover with cold salted water. Bring to the boil, then reduce the heat and simmer for 15 minutes, until soft. Drain well, then put into a large bowl with the butter and milk and season well with salt and pepper. Mash until smooth.

Preheat your oven to 190°C.

Add your peas and thyme to the mince, then transfer to a deep baking dish. Cover the lamb mixture with the mashed potatoes, then brush with the beaten egg.

Cook in your preheated oven for 40 minutes, until golden brown and bubbling.

olive oil
2 onions, diced
2 carrots, diced
2 celery sticks, diced
3 garlic cloves, finely chopped
450g lean lamb mince (5% fat or less)
2 tsp plain flour
4 tsp Worcestershire sauce
1 tsp tomato purée
1 tsp Dijon mustard
2 chicken stock cubes
450ml boiling water
salt and black pepper
60g frozen petit pois
1 tsp chopped fresh thyme

**For the mashed potato topping:**
1kg Maris Piper potatoes, peeled and chopped
25g butter
60ml low-fat milk
1 egg, beaten

## Nutritional Information

|  | Per Serving |
| --- | --- |
| Calories | 348kcal |
| Protein | 23g |
| Carbohydrates | 44g |
| Fat | 12g |

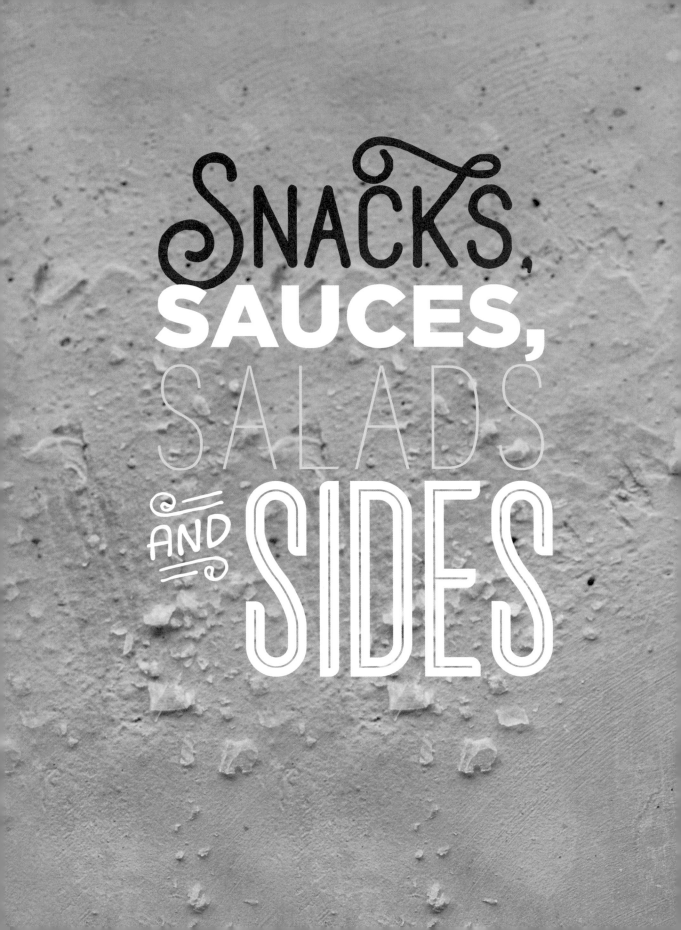

SNACKS, SAUCES, SALADS AND SIDES

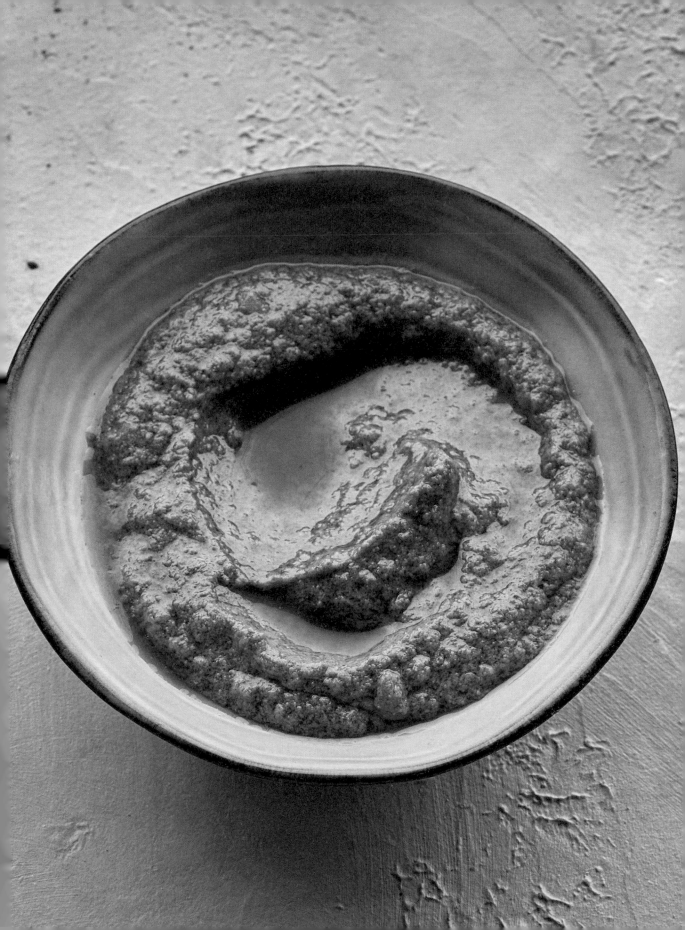

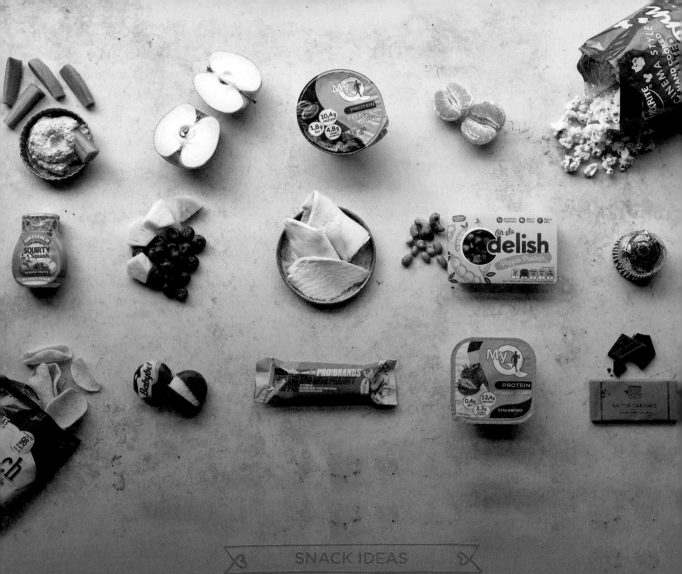

## SNACK IDEAS

**All the snacks pictured are available from Aldi**

- One small packet of baked crisps ● Fruit squash ● Carrot sticks and low-fat hummus
- Two Babybel cheeses ● Fresh blueberries and pineapple chunks ● One apple
- One protein bar ● Two slices of thinly sliced cooked turkey breast
- One pot of high-protein chocolate pudding ● One pot of high-protein quark cheese
- Aldi Oh So Delish Veggie Protein snack ● Clementine
- A few squares of dark chocolate ● One Tunnock's tea cake
- One small packet of popcorn

# GUACAMOLE

To make sure that the avocados you buy are ripe, lightly press
them – if they're soft, they are ready to rock!

⁓ ✦ —— Serves 6 —— ✦ ⁓

Scoop out your avocados into a large bowl. Add all the other
ingredients and mash until smooth.

If you store the guacamole in a tub and pop an avocado stone
in the mix, then cover the top directly with clingfilm, it should
last for up to three days in the fridge without turning black.

3 medium avocados, halved
   and stoned
1 small red onion, finely diced
1 fresh red chilli, deseeded and
   finely diced
1 lime, juiced
2 tsp olive oil
1 tsp garlic purée
salt and black pepper

**Nutritional Information**

|  | Per Serving |
|---|---|
| Calories | 186kcal |
| Protein | 3g |
| Carbohydrates | 11g |
| Fat | 14g |
| Vegetarian | ✔ |
| Gluten Free | ✔ |

# WHIPPED FETA
## WITH HONEY AND THYME

This dip is perfect served with some toasted pitta bread, spicy potato wedges (page 181) or crunchy raw vegetables. Feta is a versatile cheese that will adapt to many flavours, so don't be afraid of trying different combinations!

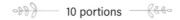 10 portions

200g feta cheese, drained

60g 0% fat Greek yoghurt

1 garlic clove, chopped

2 tbsp olive oil

1 tsp chopped fresh thyme,
   plus extra to garnish

flaky sea salt and black
   pepper

honey, for drizzling

pinch of paprika, to garnish

In a food processor, blend your feta cheese, yoghurt, garlic, olive oil and thyme. Season with black pepper.

Spoon into a bowl and drizzle with honey, then garnish with fresh thyme leaves, flaky sea salt and a light dusting of paprika. This will keep in the fridge for up to three days.

**Nutritional Information**

|  | Per Serving |
| --- | --- |
| Calories | 95kcal |
| Protein | 4g |
| Carbohydrates | 1.5g |
| Fat | 8g |
| Vegetarian | ✔ |
| Gluten Free | ✔ |

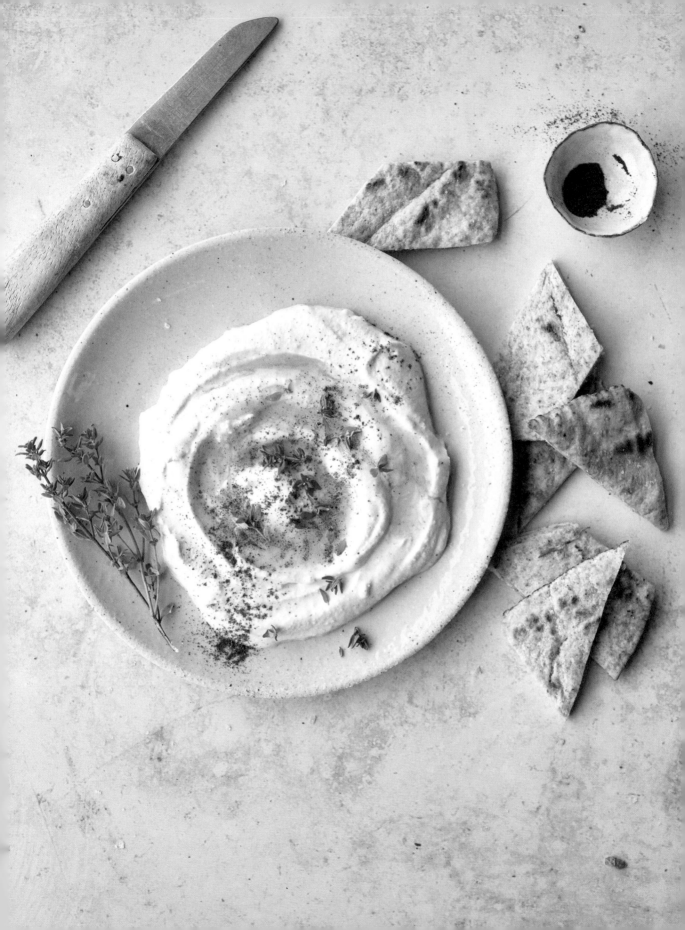

# HOMEMADE PICCALILLI

I seriously love pickles and piccalilli is one of the best. It's also class because it can last for three months in the fridge and is a great gift if you're making a hamper of food gifts. I love this with some cold meats and olives or with the pan-fried hake on page 152.

Makes 3 x 500ml jars
(50 portions)

500g cauliflower, chopped into small florets

200g courgettes, cut into large dice

100g green beans, chopped small

4 shallots, diced

2 tsp flaky sea salt

200g caster sugar

600ml white wine vinegar

3 tbsp ready-made English mustard

2 bay leaves

1 tbsp brown mustard seeds

1 tbsp coriander seeds

2 tsp cumin seeds

60g plain flour

Pop all your vegetables in a large bowl, sprinkle with the salt and set aside to marinate for 3 hours. Rinse well and pat dry.

Put your sugar, vinegar, English mustard, bay leaves and the mustard, coriander and cumin seeds in a pot and bring to a rapid boil.

Add your vegetables and the flour, then reduce the heat and simmer for 15 minutes, until your mixture thickens and your veg slightly softens.

Pour into 3 x 500ml sterilised jars and leave to cool. Put a piece of clingfilm directly on top of the pickle, then cover the jar with a lid to stop the air coming into contact with it. Store in the fridge for up to three months, checking weekly to make sure the edges of the jar are clean and that all the mix is under the clingfilm.

**Nutritional Information**

|  | Per Serving |
| --- | --- |
| Calories | 32kcal |
| Protein | 0.5g |
| Carbohydrates | 6g |
| Fat | 0.5g |
| Vegetarian | ✔ |

# SALSA VERDE

Salsa verde, or green sauce, packs a punch and adds so much depth to your meal. I love this with any fish, but a few months ago I tried it with some sirloin steak and it was perfection. Some people like to chop everything by hand, but I prefer to blend it into a smooth sauce.

—— 10 portions ——

Add everything to your blender or food processor and blitz until smooth.

The key to getting this to last for a few weeks in the fridge is to spoon it into a jar, then press a piece of clingfilm directly on top of the surface so that no air can get in and make the herbs turn black. Or to freeze this, you can pour the sauce into an ice cube tray, then, once frozen, pop the cubes out into a freezerproof bag and use as you need them.

1 shallot, chopped

4 tinned anchovies, chopped

3 garlic cloves, chopped

2 tbsp capers, drained

30g fresh flat leaf parsley (with the stalks)

30g fresh basil (with the stalks)

15g fresh mint (with the stalks – they have a lot of flavour!)

120ml extra virgin olive oil

2 tbsp white wine vinegar

1 tsp Dijon mustard

salt and black pepper

### Nutritional Information

|  | Per Serving |
| --- | --- |
| Calories | 151kcal |
| Protein | 5g |
| Carbohydrates | 3g |
| Fat | 13g |
| Gluten Free | ✔ |

# BLACK PUDDING, BLUE CHEESE, WALNUT AND APPLE SALAD

Black pudding was recently declared to be a superfood because it's high in protein and rich in iron. Black pudding is technically already cooked when you buy it, but I always recook it as I love it nice and hot. But don't be tempted to overcook it – a minute on each side is plenty just to heat it through. One of my favourite puddings is Jack McCarthy's from Kanturk in County Cork.

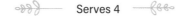 Serves 4

olive oil

175g black pudding , sliced

60g blue cheese (Cashel Blue is my favourite)

70g walnuts

1 Granny Smith apple

300g mixed baby salad leaves

**For the dressing:**

4 tsp low-fat natural yoghurt

2 tsp wholegrain mustard

2 tsp white wine vinegar

1 tsp honey

salt and black pepper

To make the dressing, put your yoghurt, mustard, vinegar, honey and some salt and pepper in a large bowl and whisk to combine. Set aside.

Heat a pan and add a little olive oil. Add the black pudding and cook on each side for 1 minute, just to seal and heat through.

Run your knife under the hot tap, then dice your blue cheese with the hot knife to cut it cleanly. Set aside.

Toast your walnuts in a hot dry pan, then tip out onto a cutting board and crush.

Grate your apple, including the skin, just before serving to prevent it from turning brown.

Place your salad leaves, black pudding, blue cheese, walnuts and apple in the bowl with the dressing and gently toss until the leaves are lightly coated, not drowned, in dressing.

Divide the salad between four bowls and serve straight away.

### Nutritional Information

|  | Per Serving |
|---|---|
| Calories | 355kcal |
| Protein | 12g |
| Carbohydrates | 18g |
| Fat | 26g |
| Vegetarian | ✔ |
| Gluten Free | ✔ |

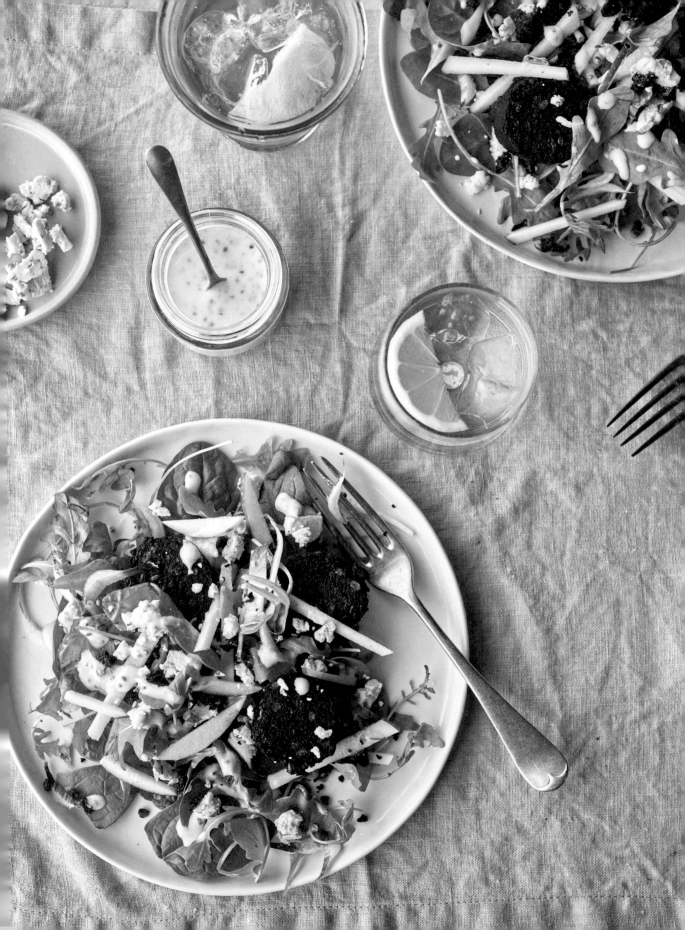

# SMOKY BACON, STRAWBERRY AND PECAN SALAD

Whenever I'm creating salads, I always remember what I learned in college: that a great salad should have more bits than leaves and that the dressing should only lightly coat the leaves, not be in a pool at the bottom of the bowl.

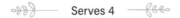 Serves 4

100g smoky bacon, chopped

40g pecan nuts, crushed

500g mixed leaves (lambs' lettuce, red chard, rocket and spinach)

1 punnet of strawberries, hulled and quartered

1 red onion, thinly sliced

**For the dressing:**

40g low-fat natural yoghurt

2 tbsp red wine vinegar

1 tbsp olive oil

salt and pepper

Heat a frying pan and add your chopped bacon (you don't need to add any oil). Cook until the fat has rendered out of the bacon, then add your bashed pecan nuts and cook until the nuts are toasted and the bacon is crisp. Drain on a plate lined with kitchen paper to remove the excess oil.

Put your natural yoghurt, red wine vinegar, olive oil and some salt and pepper in a jam jar, then screw on the lid and shake to combine.

Put the salad leaves in a large bowl with the bacon, pecans, strawberries and red onion. Just before serving, add your dressing and toss to coat your leaves.

Divide between four bowls and serve straight away.

**Nutritional Information**

|  | Per Serving |
| --- | --- |
| Calories | 279kcal |
| Protein | 11g |
| Carbohydrates | 13g |
| Fat | 19g |
| Gluten Free | ✔ |

# SPICY POTATO WEDGES

These remind me of my childhood, running into the shop for some wedges on a Friday.

Serves 3

Preheat your oven to 240°C.

Rinse your potato wedges under cold running water to remove the starch, then pat dry with a clean tea towel.

Place in a bowl, then add your oil, spices and some salt and pepper and mix well to make sure all the wedges are coated. Place on a baking tray in a single layer, making sure they aren't piled on top of one other.

Cook in the preheated oven for 15 minutes, then take the tray out of the oven and turn over all the wedges. Return to the oven and cook for another 30 minutes.

4 Maris Piper potatoes,
   unpeeled and cut into
   wedges
2 tsp olive oil
1 tsp cayenne pepper
1 tsp garlic powder
1 tsp paprika
salt and black pepper

**Nutritional Information**

|  | Per Serving |
| --- | --- |
| Calories | 205kcal |
| Protein | 4g |
| Carbohydrates | 37g |
| Fat | 4g |
| Vegetarian | ✔ |
| Gluten Free | ✔ |

# CAPRESE SALAD

Sometimes salads involve a fair bit of work to taste good, which is why I adore this salad – it's so quick and easy to make. The hardest thing you have to do is season it well. It always reminds me of holidays with my friend Laura. As soon as we are off the plane, we have a Caprese salad in front of us!

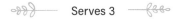 Serves 3

3 large ripe tomatoes, thinly sliced

salt and black pepper

3 balls of fresh mozzarella, thinly sliced

10 fresh basil leaves

1 tbsp olive oil

1 tsp balsamic vinegar

Season your tomato slices with salt and pepper, then arrange your mozzarella and tomatoes in alternate slices on a serving platter. Tear your basil all over the top.

Whisk your olive oil and vinegar together to make your dressing and season with salt and pepper, then drizzle lightly over the top of the salad.

**Nutritional Information**

|  | Per Serving |
|---|---|
| Calories | 205kcal |
| Protein | 11g |
| Carbohydrates | 6g |
| Fat | 15g |
| Vegetarian | ✔ |
| Gluten Free | ✔ |

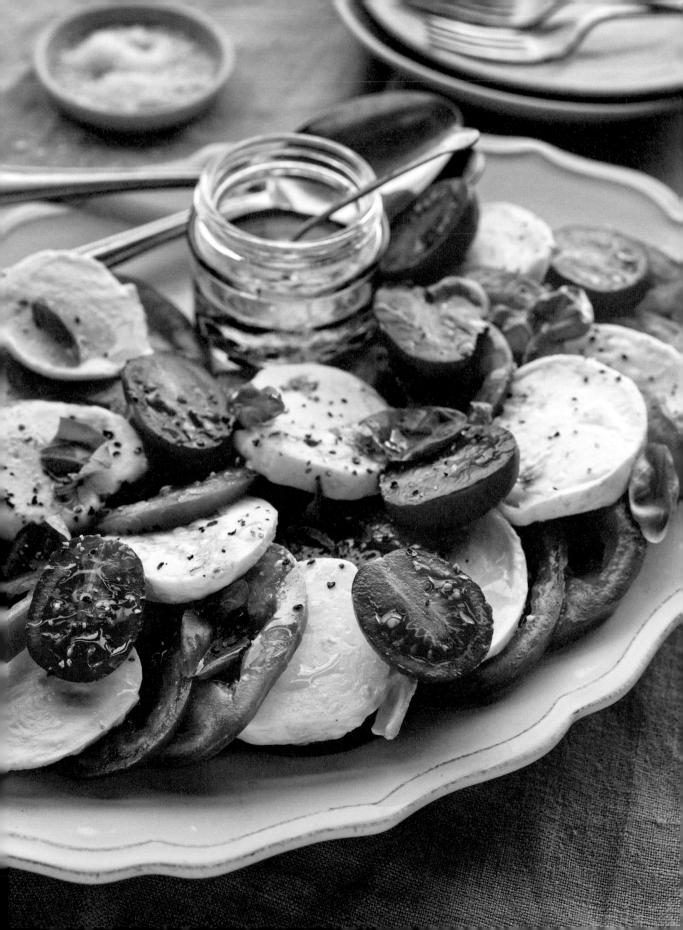

# CURRIED COCONUT POTATOES

This is a gorgeous side dish that's suitable for vegans. You can even have these on their own.
I love making this in the summer but the potato that I use all year round is Maris Piper,
as it's a dry, floury potato that's delicious.

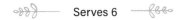 Serves 6

6 Maris Piper potatoes

1 lemongrass stick

olive oil

2 shallots, chopped

3 garlic cloves, chopped

2.5cm piece of fresh ginger, peeled
    and grated

1 fresh red chilli, deseeded and finely
    chopped (reserve some for garnish)

1 tbsp curry powder

2 tsp ground turmeric

1 x 400ml tin of low-fat coconut milk

2 limes, juiced

2 spring onions, thinly sliced

handful of fresh coriander, chopped
    (reserve some for garnish)

Parboil your potatoes for 10 minutes, then drain and
leave to cool.

Using a heavy pan, bash your lemongrass on a cutting
board, then finely chop it.

Heat a wide frying pan and add some oil. Add your
lemongrass, shallots, garlic, ginger, chilli, curry powder
and turmeric and cook for 1 minute, then stir in your
coconut milk and simmer for a few more minutes.

Slice your cooled potatoes into discs, then add to the
coconut milk mixture. Simmer for 10 minutes.

Stir in your lime juice, spring onions and coriander.
Garnish with the reserved red chilli and coriander and
serve hot.

**Nutritional Information**

|  | Per Serving |
| --- | --- |
| Calories | 273kcal |
| Protein | 5g |
| Carbohydrates | 34g |
| Fat | 13g |
| Vegetarian | ✔ |
| Gluten Free | ✔ |

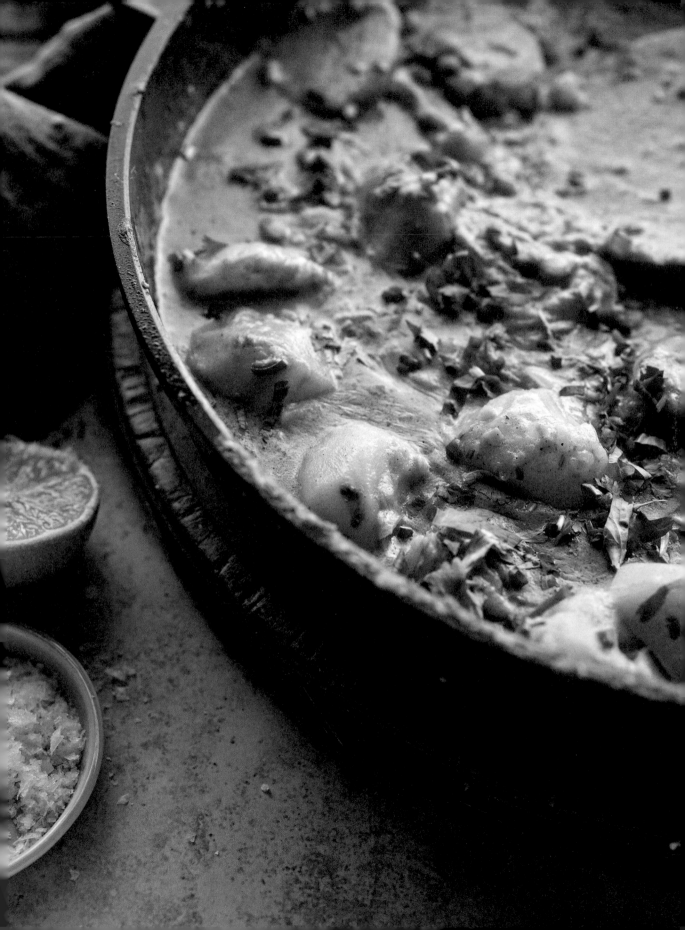

# GARLIC AND ROSEMARY MASHED POTATOES

You can really overload the calories in mashed potatoes, so just do some cute swaps and use light cream and light milk. The key to a good mash is to make sure your potatoes are well drained and dried out. If you would like a plain mash, then just leave out the rosemary and garlic. When seasoning mash, use white pepper instead of black pepper so the mash doesn't have black specks in it.

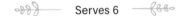 Serves 6

2kg Maris Piper potatoes, peeled and cut into large cubes

60g butter

150ml low-fat milk

100ml light cream

6 garlic cloves, left unpeeled and whole but bashed

3 sprigs of fresh rosemary (reserve some for garnish)

salt and white pepper

Put your potatoes in a large pot and cover with cold salted water. Bring to the boil, then reduce the heat and cook for 25 minutes, until softened. Pierce the potatoes with a knife to check. Drain in a colander and leave to drain in the sink for 5 minutes to make sure all the excess water is drained off.

Place your butter, milk, cream, garlic and rosemary in a small pot. Simmer for 5 minutes to melt the butter and let the flavours infuse, then strain off your rosemary and garlic.

Mash your potatoes before you add your liquid. If you have a NutriBullet, it's so handy to pop in the cooked spuds and blitz any lumps out. Don't add all the liquid in one go, as you can always add more but you can't take it out if you add too much! Mix well, then season with salt and white pepper. Garnish with a small sprig of rosemary on top and serve hot.

## Nutritional Information

|  | Per Serving |
|---|---|
| Calories | 390kcal |
| Protein | 9g |
| Carbohydrates | 61g |
| Fat | 11g |
| Vegetarian | ✔ |
| Gluten Free | ✔ |

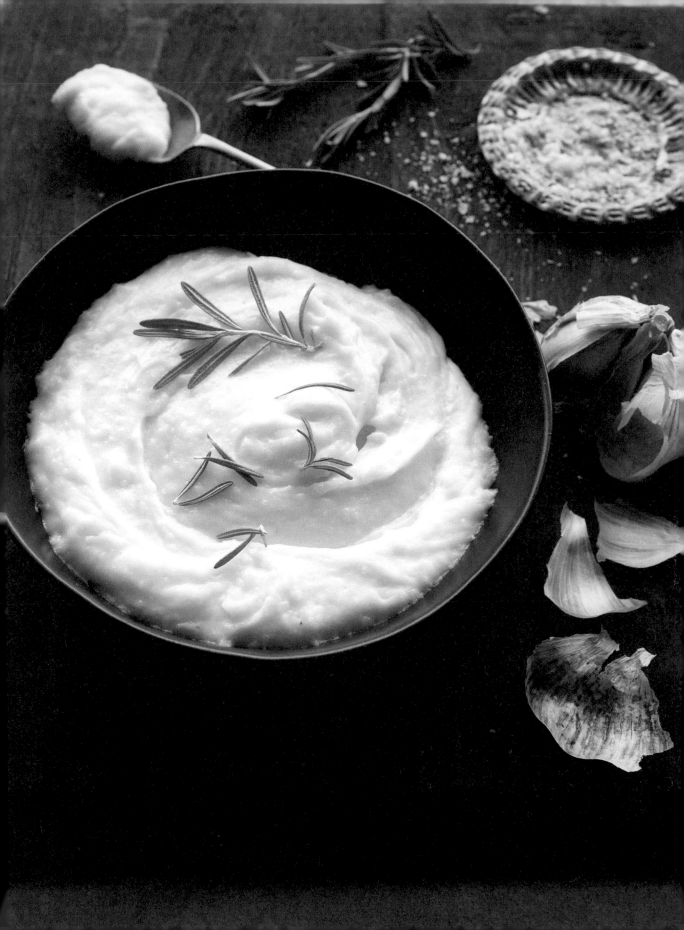

# HASSELBACK POTATOES

Now I may be sounding like the most Irish person ever, but I think spuds are class. I love how versatile one vegetable can be and how many variations you can get from it. These bad boys are insane. They're like a cross between a pack of crisps and a roast potato! You can go as thick or as thin as you want with the slices, but I prefer a thinner slice. Always try to use Maris Pipers, as they work the best here since they're a drier spud.

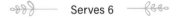 Serves 6

6 large Maris Piper
   potatoes, unpeeled
olive oil
salt and black pepper
1 bunch of fresh chives,
   finely chopped

Preheat your oven to 200°C.

Using a sharp knife, cut thin slices across the potato, going straight down but without cutting the whole way through. You want each potato to have lots of thin slices but still be held together at the bottom.

Place the potatoes on a large baking tray and drizzle your olive oil over each potato, then season with salt and pepper. Roast in the preheated oven for 60 minutes.

To serve, scatter your chopped chives over the top.

**Nutritional Information**

|  | Per Serving |
| --- | --- |
| Calories | 155kcal |
| Protein | 4g |
| Carbohydrates | 28g |
| Fat | 3g |
| Vegetarian | ✔ |
| Gluten Free | ✔ |

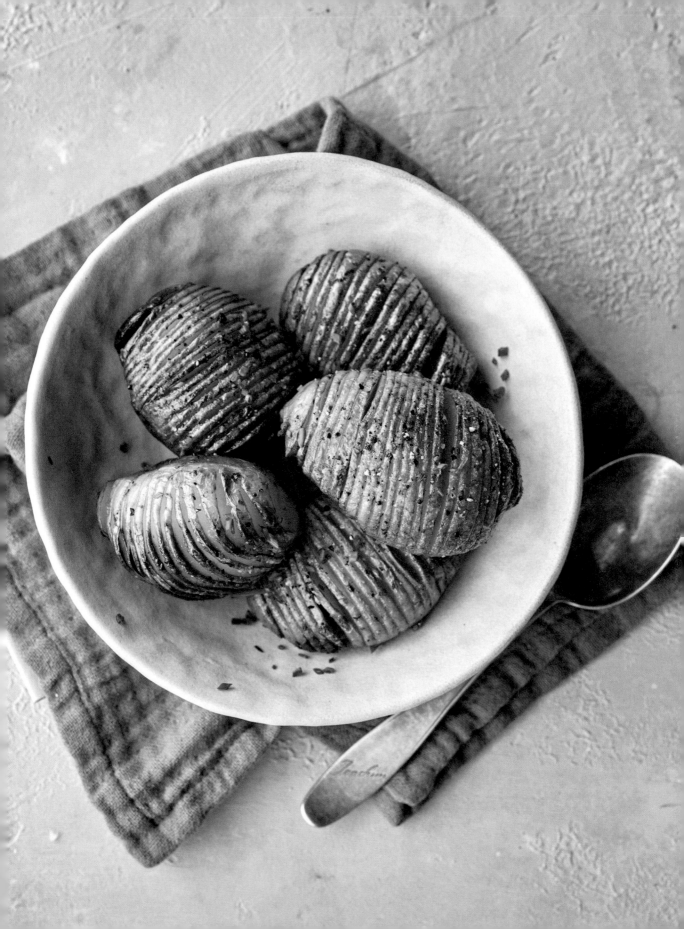

# SPICY CAULIFLOWER 'WINGS'

This is a vegan version of buffalo chicken wings. They can be served with a simple sauce but I adore these on a bed of fluffy basmati rice with some chopped spring onions and red chilli on top. It's budget friendly but a bit high in calories, so make it only now and then as a special treat.

Serves 2

100g plain flour

150ml water

1 tbsp light soy sauce

1 tbsp sesame seeds

1 small cauliflower, broken into bite-sized florets

40g dried breadcrumbs (panko are the best here)

boiled basmati rice, to serve

2 spring onions, thinly sliced, to garnish

1 fresh red chilli, deseeded and thinly sliced, to garnish

fresh coriander leaves, to garnish

**For the sauce:**

60g chilli purée

2 garlic cloves, minced

2.5cm piece of fresh ginger, peeled and grated

15g light brown sugar

1 tbsp rice vinegar

1 tbsp sesame oil

Preheat your oven to 200°C.

Put the flour, water, soy sauce and sesame seeds in a large bowl and whisk into a batter. Add your cauliflower florets and stir to coat, then sprinkle in your breadcrumbs and stir again until all the florets are coated with crumbs.

Place on a baking tray in a single layer, making sure the florets aren't piled on top of one another. Roast in the preheated oven for 20–25 minutes, until golden brown. I shake the tray after 10 minutes to get them moving.

Meanwhile, to make the sauce, whisk together your chilli purée, garlic, ginger, brown sugar, rice vinegar and sesame oil in a large bowl.

Once the florets are done, take them out of the oven and pop them in the sauce. Toss them around in the bowl to coat them all.

Serve with boiled basmati rice and scatter the spring onions, chilli and coriander on top.

**Nutritional Information**

|  | Per Serving |
|---|---|
| Calories | 539kcal |
| Protein | 16g |
| Carbohydrates | 84g |
| Fat | 15g |
| Vegetarian | ✔ |

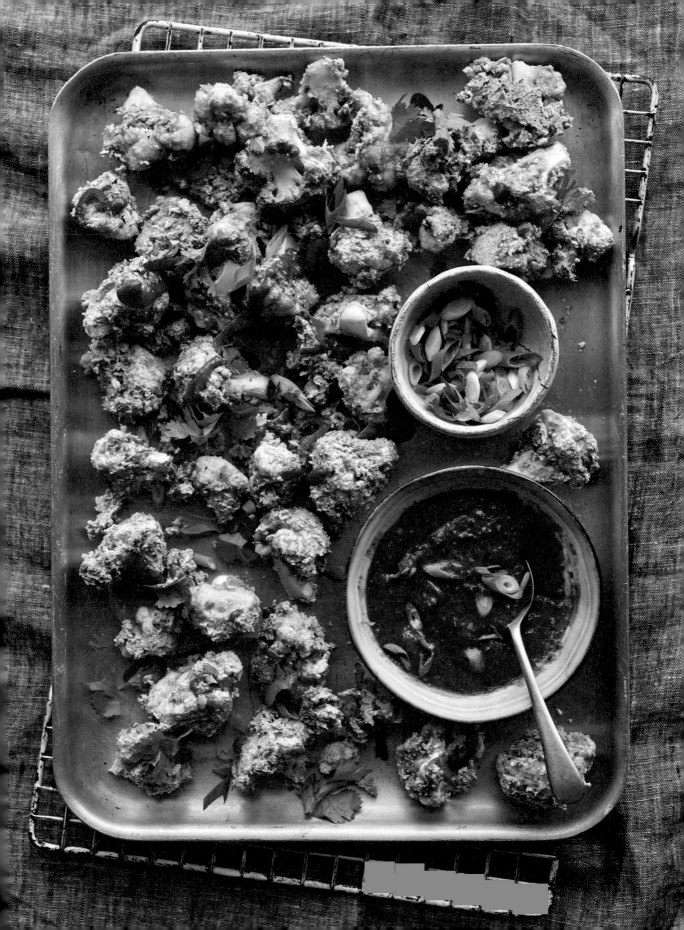

# BRAISED MARINATED ONIONS

I adore onions. I think they're amazing cooked or raw, but when you marinate them it mellows out their strong flavour. This is such a simple side that would go well with roast beef (page 128) or a steak dinner. Sometimes the usual vegetables can be boring, but I think most households have onions in the press! I leave the skin on these so that they hold their shape, but don't worry, once they're cooked you can easily slip off the skins before eating them.

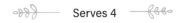 Serves 4

40g light brown sugar

3 garlic cloves, chopped

1 tsp chilli flakes

200ml water

200ml red wine vinegar

4 white onions, unpeeled and cut in half across the middle

50g butter, cut into 8 cubes

salt and black pepper

4 sprigs of fresh rosemary, chopped, plus extra to garnish

Mix together your brown sugar, garlic, chilli flakes, water and red wine vinegar in a roasting tray. Put the onions in the tray, cut side down. Cover the tray with clingfilm and marinate in the fridge for at least 4 hours or overnight.

Preheat your oven to 200°C.

Flip the onions upside down so that the cut side is now facing up. Place a knob of butter on top of each onion half, then season with salt and pepper and scatter your rosemary on top of each onion.

Roast in the preheated oven, uncovered, for 1 hour, until they have softened and caramelised and are golden brown. Garnish with extra rosemary and serve hot.

**Nutritional Information**

|  | Per Serving |
| --- | --- |
| Calories | 190kcal |
| Protein | 2g |
| Carbohydrates | 22g |
| Fat | 10g |
| Vegetarian | ✔ |
| Gluten Free | ✔ |

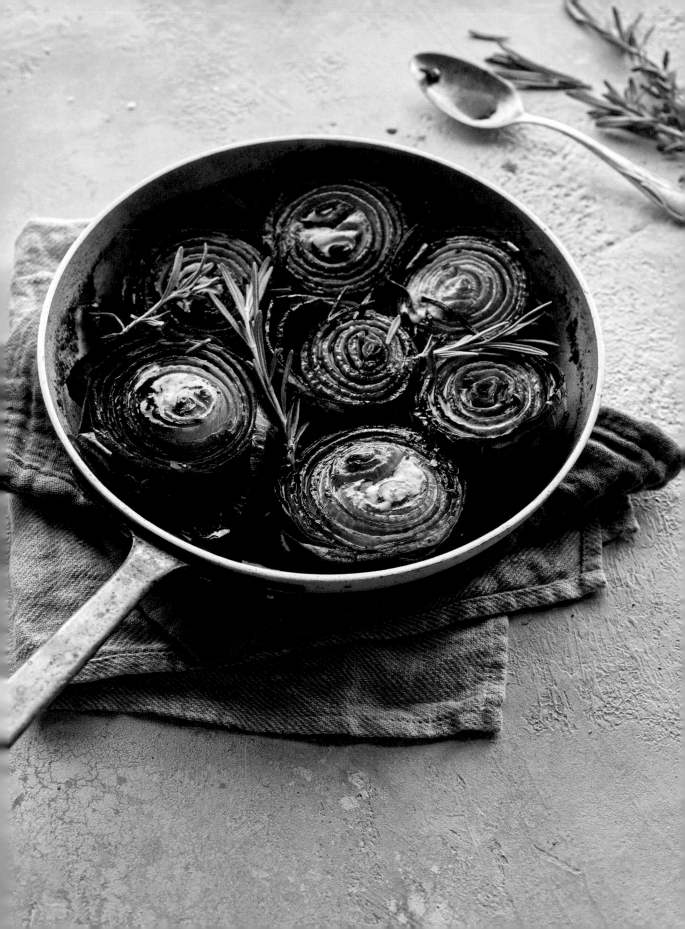

# CHEESY CAULIFLOWER

A classic combination and a perfect side to round out a roast dinner on a Sunday. This dish can be made the night before, then finished in the oven the next day.

Serves 3

1 large cauliflower, chopped
    into florets
olive oil
1 white onion, diced
50g butter
30g plain flour
450ml low-fat milk
1 bay leaf
salt and white pepper
40g light Cheddar cheese,
    grated

Preheat your oven to 180°C.

Place a pot of water on to boil. Once the water is boiling rapidly, pop in your cauliflower. As soon as it comes back up to the boil, drain your cauliflower and set aside.

Heat a saucepan and add your olive oil. Add your onion and gently sauté until softened. Add your butter and flour and cook for a couple of minutes to create a roux (this will thicken your sauce).

Pour in your milk and whisk until smooth, with no lumps of roux left, then add your bay leaf. Season with salt and white pepper and simmer for 5 minutes, stirring often.

Place your cauliflower florets in a baking dish, then pour over your white sauce and top with the grated cheese. Bake in the preheated oven for 30 minutes, until golden brown on top. Serve hot.

## Nutritional Information

|  | Per Serving |
| --- | --- |
| Calories | 300kcal |
| Protein | 11g |
| Carbohydrates | 30g |
| Fat | 15g |
| Vegetarian | ✔ |

# SAUTÉED MUSHROOMS COOKED IN A TOFU MOUSSE

This is an amazing vegan side dish, as spinach is packed full of iron, vitamin D and other nutrients. I know it seems like a load of spinach, but don't worry, it will wilt down. I like to serve this with some pan-fried seabass or grilled halloumi.

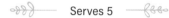 Serves 5

Blitz your tofu, soy sauce, mirin and rice wine vinegar in a NutriBullet or food processor until smooth.

Heat a frying pan and add some olive oil, then add your mushrooms, garlic and ginger. Cook until the mushrooms have softened and shrunk, then drain off the excess liquid.

Add your tofu mousse and cook until warmed through. Add your spinach and season well with salt and pepper.

Plate up the mushrooms and tofu mousse and serve immediately.

200g silken tofu

60ml light soy sauce

2 tbsp mirin

2 tbsp rice wine vinegar

olive oil

200g wild mushrooms

4 garlic cloves, chopped

2.5cm piece of fresh ginger, peeled and grated

300g spinach

salt and black pepper

### Nutritional Information

|  | Per Serving |
|---|---|
| Calories | 192kcal |
| Protein | 8g |
| Carbohydrates | 14g |
| Fat | 11g |
| Vegetarian | ✔ |

# ROASTED MEDITERRANEAN VEGETABLES
## WITH GARLIC AND THYME

One of my favourite dinners is chicken, potato wedges and these veg. If you have some pesto, pop a dollop on top – it's divine! This is also a great vegetarian main course on a bed of cous-cous with some feta crumbled on top. You can roast any sturdy vegetables – just toss them in olive oil and roast away. Roasting vegetables helps to deepen the flavour. Thyme works well but rosemary, basil and oregano are also delicious.

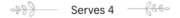 Serves 4

4 red onions, cut into wedges

3 red peppers, cut into large chunky pieces

4 garlic cloves, sliced

1 courgette, sliced

12 cherry tomatoes

2 tbsp extra virgin olive oil

6 sprigs of fresh thyme

salt and black pepper

Preheat your oven to 200°C.

Place all your vegetables in a roasting tray and drizzle over your olive oil, then scatter your thyme on top and season with salt and pepper. Time to get your hands dirty! Massage the oil into the vegetables so that they are evenly covered in oil and seasoning.

Pop into the oven for 30 minutes. Remove from the oven and shake up the tray to move the vegetables around, then roast for a further 15 minutes. Serve hot.

**Nutritional Information**

|  | Per Serving |
| --- | --- |
| Calories | 134kcal |
| Protein | 4g |
| Carbohydrates | 12g |
| Fat | 7g |
| Vegetarian | ✔ |
| Gluten Free | ✔ |

# ASPARAGUS WRAPPED IN TURKEY RASHERS
## WITH A LEMON DIP

Asparagus is best when it's in season in May and June, when it's at its sweetest. This is a classic dish that can be enjoyed as nibbles in front of the telly or as part of a dinner party. The turkey rashers are lower in calories than your traditional Parma ham and full of protein. I've also swapped the sauce from a traditional beurre blanc to save on the calories.

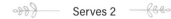 Serves 2

Put a pot of water on to boil and add some salt to it. To prep the asparagus, trim the ends 2.5cm up from the bottom, as this part is usually very woody and hard to chew. Blanch your asparagus in the boiling water for 2 minutes, then drain and refresh under cold running water.

Wrap a piece of turkey rasher around each asparagus spear.

Heat a frying pan and add the olive oil. Add the asparagus spears and cook until the rashers are golden brown. Season with salt and pepper.

To make your dip, simply combine your yoghurt, shallot, chives and lemon juice, then spoon into two ramekins. Serve the asparagus spears with the ramekin on the side for dipping.

10 asparagus spears
5 turkey rashers, cut in half
1 tsp olive oil
salt and black pepper

**For the lemon dip:**
100g low-fat natural or
    Greek yoghurt
1 shallot, finely diced
1 tsp chopped fresh chives
squeeze of lemon juice

## Nutritional Information

| | Per Serving |
|---|---|
| Calories | 200kcal |
| Protein | 25g |
| Carbohydrates | 7g |
| Fat | 8g |
| Gluten Free | ✔ |

# BRAISED RED CABBAGE

When we think of vegetables we often think boring and bland, but winter vegetables are just incredible. All they need is some TLC and they will burst with flavour.

—— Serves 3 ——

1 head of red cabbage

70g light brown sugar

60g butter

150ml red wine

1 cinnamon stick

1 red onion, sliced

Quarter the cabbage and remove the core, then shred. Put your sugar, butter, red wine and cinnamon stick in a pot and bring to a simmer. Add your cabbage and red onion and pop a lid on top to braise.

Gently cook on a low heat, stirring occasionally, for 75 minutes. Serve hot.

**Nutritional Information**

|  | Per Serving |
|---|---|
| Calories | 298kcal |
| Protein | 4g |
| Carbohydrates | 32g |
| Fat | 17g |
| Vegetarian | ✔ |
| Gluten Free | ✔ |

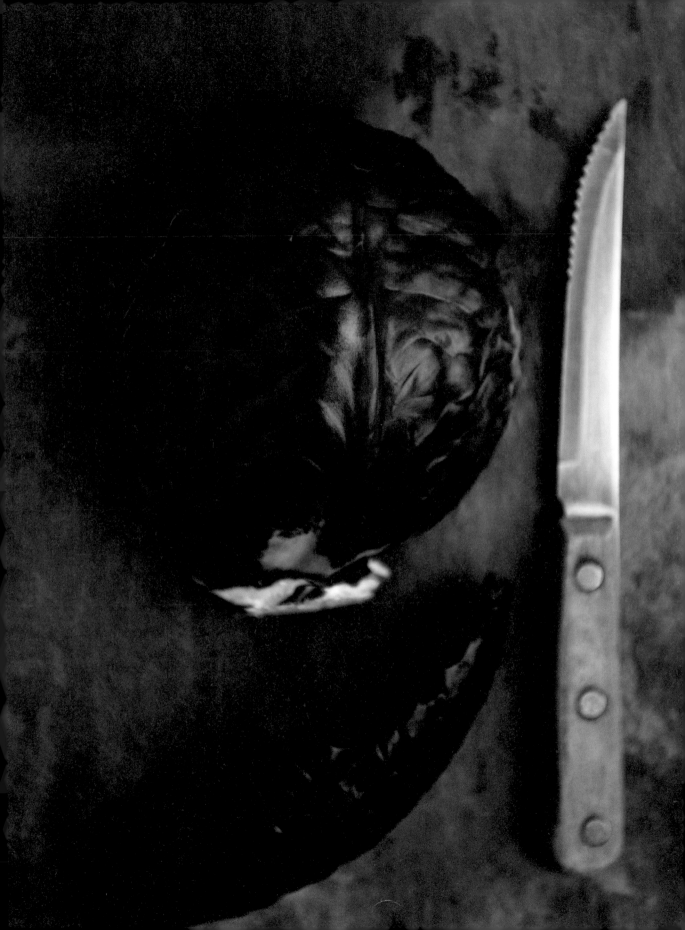

# Treats
## and
## Desserts

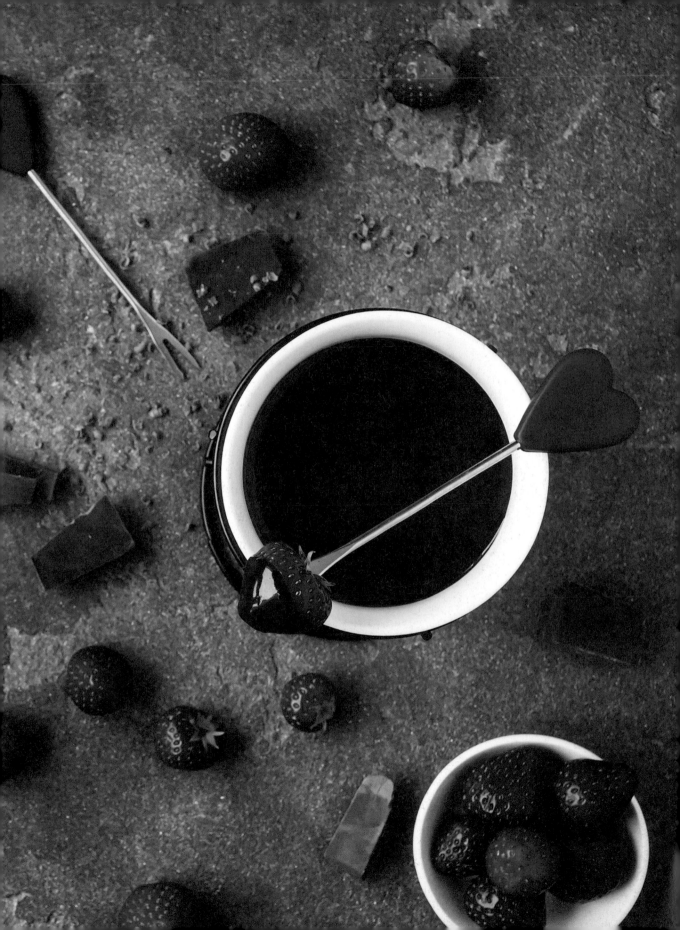

# BANANA BREAD

We all went a bit mad on banana bread during the first COVID-19 lockdown in Ireland, so this recipe has been tried and tested many times in the Lewis household! This is delicious but be careful with the portion control. Make sure you implement some discipline and have two slices max with a mug of hot tea.

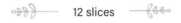 12 slices

250g self-raising flour
140g brown sugar
1 tsp ground cinnamon
3 over-ripe bananas, mashed
3 eggs, beaten
150g butter, melted

Preheat your oven to 170°C. Grease 2 x 1lb loaf tins.
Mix your flour, brown sugar and cinnamon in a large bowl.

In a separate bowl, mix together your mashed bananas, eggs and butter. Add this to the flour mixture and mix well.

Pour into your two greased tins and bake in the preheated oven for 90 minutes.

Cool on a wire rack, then cut each loaf into six slices.

**Nutritional Information**

|  | Per Serving |
|---|---|
| Calories | 255kcal |
| Protein | 4g |
| Carbohydrates | 34g |
| Fat | 11g |
| Vegetarian | ✔ |

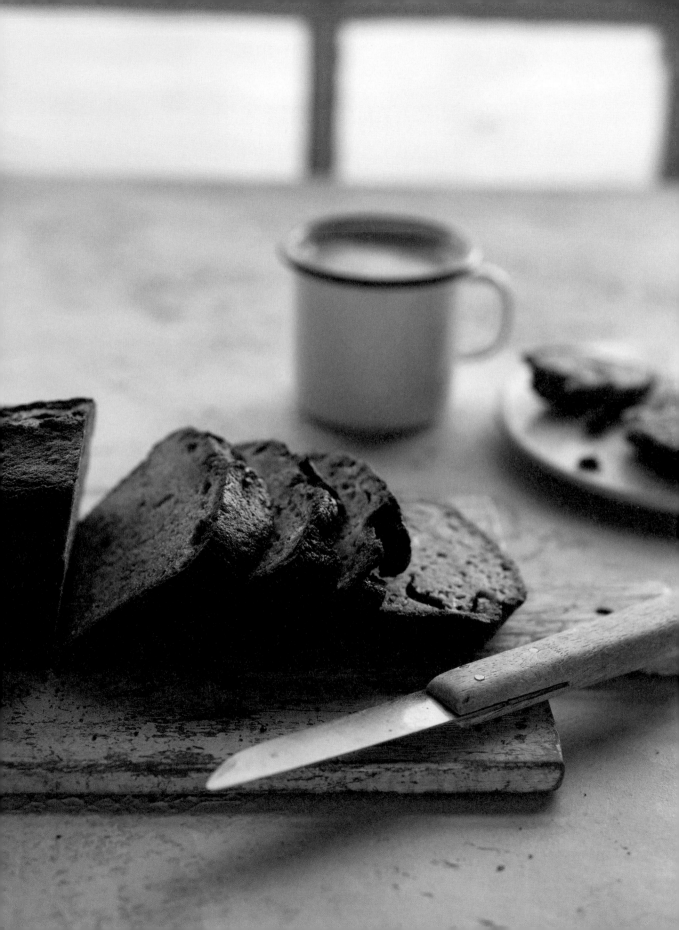

# STRAWBERRY JAM AND OAT CAKES

These could technically go into the breakfast chapter, but I think we need to be realistic and slot this into treats. If you eat too many you could break your calorie balance, so behave! These are so good with a cup of tea. You can have them at room temperature but personally I love them directly from the fridge.

16 portions

125g plain flour
100g butter, diced and at room temperature
95g oats
80g stevia or Canderel sweetener
80g toasted pecan nuts, chopped
2 tsp honey
1 large egg
100g strawberry jam

Preheat your oven to 180°C. Line a 20cm square brownie tin with non-stick baking paper.

Put all your ingredients except the jam in a blender or food processor and blitz to combine.

Spread half of the dough on the baking tray, then spread your jam in the middle, going all the way to the edges, and top with the remaining dough.

Bake in the preheated oven for 35 minutes. Allow to cool on a wire rack before cutting into 16 squares. Store in an airtight container in the fridge.

**Nutritional Information**

|  | Per Serving |
|---|---|
| Calories | 161kcal |
| Protein | 2.5g |
| Carbohydrates | 15g |
| Fat | 10g |
| Vegetarian | ✔ |

# BERRY, CINNAMON AND ORANGE COMPOTE

This is so handy to have in the fridge in a jar. This can be used on top of toasted coconut bread (page 104), porridge or yoghurt.

Serves 2

Put your orange juice and brown sugar in a saucepan and bring to the boil. Add your berries, orange zest and cinnamon stick, then reduce the heat and gently simmer until the berries are softened but still holding their shape.

Place in a jar and leave to cool. Store in your fridge, covered with a lid. If you put a piece of clingfilm directly on top of the surface of the compote, it will keep for even longer.

50g light brown sugar
1 orange, zested and juiced
200g frozen mixed berries
1 cinnamon stick

## Nutritional Information

|  | Per Serving |
|---|---|
| Calories | 175kcal |
| Protein | 2g |
| Carbohydrates | 37g |
| Fat | 2g |
| Vegetarian | ✔ |
| Gluten Free | ✔ |

# ORANGE OAT FLAPJACKS

These are just so delicious as a snack or a quick breakfast on the go. I'm a big fan of oats as they keep you nice and full since they're high in fibre and give you slow-releasing energy. These are so easy to make and can be popped into the kids' lunchboxes as a nice treat for them, but you still know they're getting a good source of fibre.

— 15 portions —

110g butter, plus extra for greasing
75g light brown sugar
3 tbsp honey
270g oats
2 oranges, zested

Preheat your oven to 190°C. Grease a 20cm square tin with a little butter.

Melt the butter, brown sugar and honey in a large saucepan, then stir in your oats and orange zest. Pour out onto the greased tray, making sure it's even and flat. Bake in the preheated oven for 18 minutes.

Allow to cool on a wire rack, then cut into 15 slices and keep in an airtight container. I always keep mine in the fridge because it makes them nice and chewy, but that's just my personal preference.

**Nutritional Information**

|  | Per Serving |
| --- | --- |
| Calories | 151kcal |
| Protein | 2g |
| Carbohydrates | 19g |
| Fat | 7g |
| Vegetarian | ✔ |

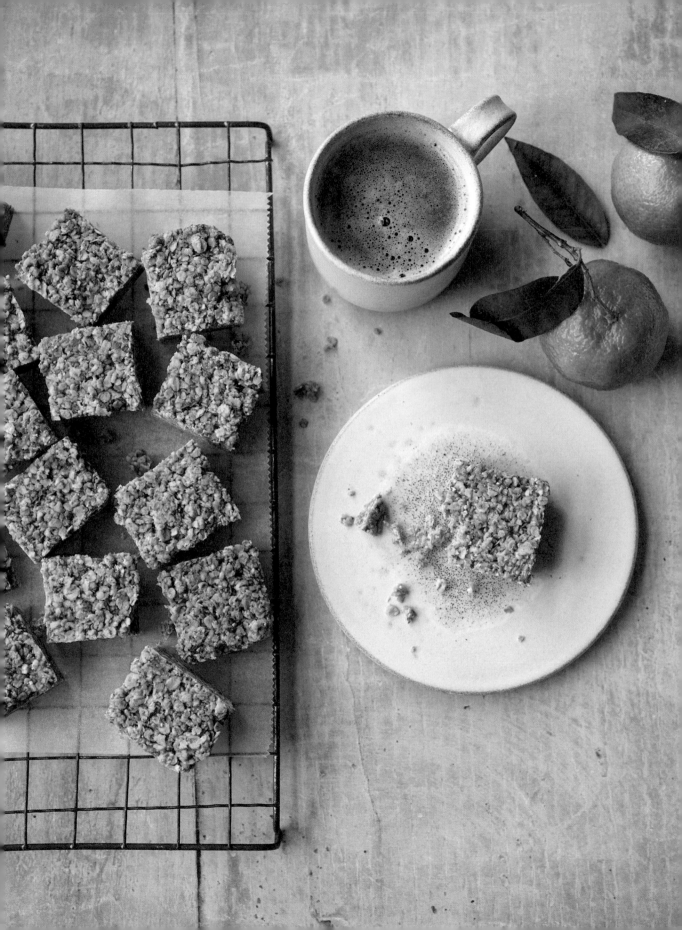

# CHOCOLATE POTS
## WITH FRESH RASPBERRIES

These are that little hit of sweetness that you may need if you're craving a treat. The key is to have just the one! They are so simple and can be whipped up in a few minutes.

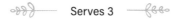 Serves 3

80g dark chocolate, finely
    chopped (70% cocoa
    solids is the best)
120ml full-fat cream
2 tsp vanilla extract
fresh raspberries, to serve
fresh mint, to serve

Melt your chocolate in a bowl. Add your cream and vanilla extract and stir to combine, then divide the mixture between three ramekins.

Cover the ramekins with clingfilm and refrigerate for 2 hours.

Serve with fresh raspberries and a tiny sprig of fresh mint and enjoy with a cup of tea.

## Nutritional Information

|  | Per Serving |
| --- | --- |
| Calories | 300kcal |
| Protein | 4g |
| Carbohydrates | 10g |
| Fat | 26g |
| Vegetarian | ✔ |

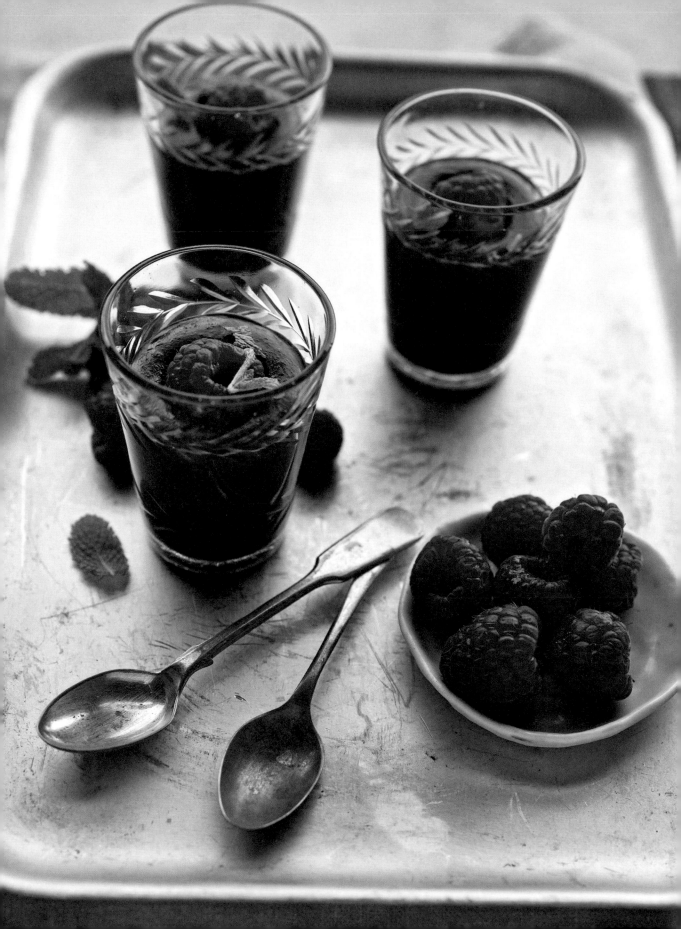

# SALTED PEANUT BUTTER FROZEN YOGHURT

Sometimes all you crave is ice cream. You might remember from my first book that I love Snickers ice cream, so I just had to figure out a way to get that same flavour hit (especially if you add an extra drizzle of peanut butter and some roasted peanuts on top). You can enjoy this without overindulging on the calories that regular ice cream is full of.

Serves 8

800g low-fat natural yoghurt
100g peanut butter
40g stevia or Canderel sweetener
1 tsp flaky sea salt
espresso shots, to serve (optional)

Freeze your yoghurt. Once it's frozen, put it in your NutriBullet, high-speed blender or food processor along with your peanut butter and sweetener and blitz to combine.

Place back in the freezer in an airtight freezerproof container and sprinkle the flaky sea salt evenly over the top. Leave for 4 hours or more.

Enjoy with a shot of espresso on top if you like.

**Nutritional Information**

|  | Per Serving |
| --- | --- |
| Calories | 181kcal |
| Protein | 11g |
| Carbohydrates | 11g |
| Fat | 10g |
| Vegetarian | ✔ |
| Gluten Free | ✔ |

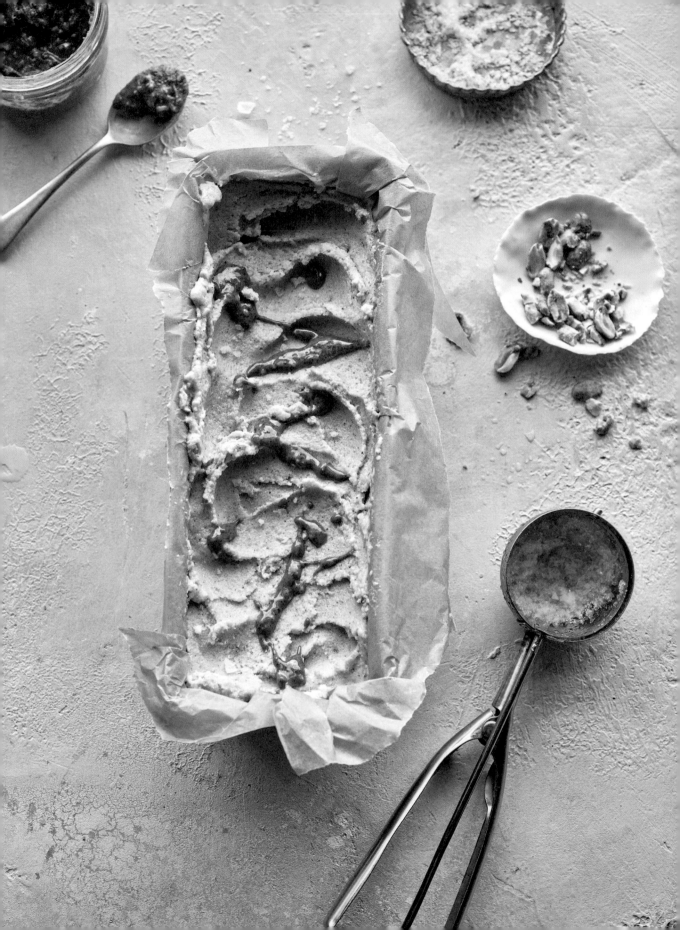

# STEWED APPLE
## WITH NATURAL YOGHURT AND CINNAMON

Sometimes something traditional and simple is exactly what you need.
My nana would always make this for us. Sometimes she served it with ice cream,
but that's not ideal for weight loss, so I have it with yoghurt now instead.

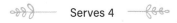 Serves 4

4 cooking apples, such as
   Bramley apples, peeled,
   cored and chopped
400ml Diet 7up
800g low-fat natural
   yoghurt
pinch of ground cinnamon,
   to serve

Place your apples in a large saucepan with your Diet
7up and simmer until they have softened. Remove the
pan from the heat and allow to cool, then store in your
fridge.

To serve, spoon the stewed apple on top of your
yoghurt, like a compote, and top with a pinch of
cinnamon.

**Nutritional Information**

|  | Per Serving |
| --- | --- |
| Calories | 340kcal |
| Protein | 9g |
| Carbohydrates | 33g |
| Fat | 19g |
| Vegetarian | ✔ |
| Gluten Free | ✔ |

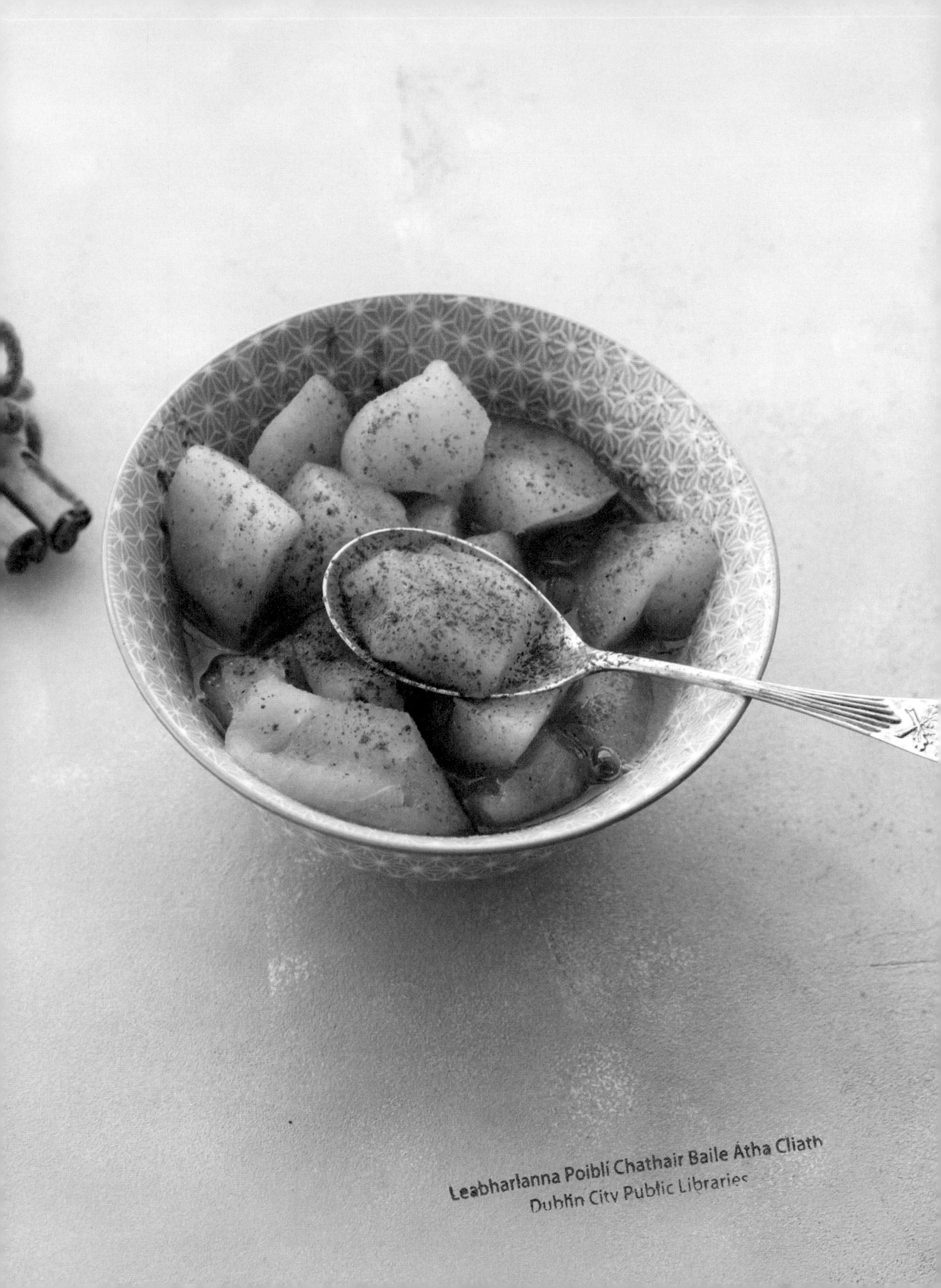

# INDEX

# NOTES

# NOTES

# NOTES

# NOTES

# NOTES

# NOTES

# NOTES